ANAESTHESIA FOR THE HIGH RISK PATIENT

ANAESTHESIA FOR THE HIGH RISK PATIENT

Edited by
Dr Ian McConachie, *Consultant in Anaesthesia & Intensive Care*
Blackpool Victoria Hospital

© 2002

Greenwich Medical Media Limited
137 Euston Road
London NW1 2AA

870 Market Street, Ste 720,
San Francisco, CA 94102

ISBN 1 84110 072 2

First Published 2002

A catalogue record for this book is available from the British Library.

Project Manager
Gavin Smith

Typeset by Charon Tec Pvt. Ltd, Chennai, India

Printed by Ashford Colour Press Ltd, Hants

Distributed by Plymbridge Distributors Ltd and
in the USA by Jamco Distribution

Visit our website at **www.greenwich-medical.co.uk**

CONTENTS

Preface vii

Contributors ix

1. Epidemiology and identification of the high-risk surgical patient 1
   A. Adams

2. Respiratory risk and complications 29
   A. Adams

3. Lessons from the National Confidential Enquiry into
   Perioperative Deaths 41
   K. Paramesh and C. Dunkley

4. Analgesia for the high risk patient 51
   F. Duncan and D.J. Counsell

5. Local anaesthetic techniques 65
   B. Lord

6. The critically ill patient in the operating theatre 77
   D. Hume and I. McConachie

7. The elderly patient 101
   S. Vaughan

8. Perioperative optimisation 117
   M. Cutts

9. The patient with coronary heart disease 127
   S. Lakshmanan and M. Hartley

10. Valvular heart disease and pulmonary hypertension 141
    C. Harle

11. Emergency abdominal aortic surgery 153
    G. Johnson and M. Chamberlain

12. Gastrointestinal surgery 165
    A. Heard and N. Harper

13. Perioperative renal insufficiency and failure 179
    I. McConachie

14. The role of the cardiology consult 199
    S. Bulugahapitiya and D. Hesketh Roberts

15. The risk of anaemia and blood transfusion 215
    M. Bewsher

16. Admission criteria for HDU and ICU 227
    V. Prasad and J. Cupitt

17. The meaning of risk 239
    A. Adams

Index 249

PREFACE

This text:

- Is aimed primarily at trainees in Anaesthesia though more experienced practitioners may find it useful as a refresher in recent concepts and advances. A basic knowledge of physiology, pharmacology and anaesthesia is assumed.

- May be a useful '*aide memoire*' for the FRCA and other examinations in anaesthesia.

- Aims to provide practical information on the management of high-risk patients presenting for surgery as well as sufficient background information to enable understanding of the principles and rationale behind their anaesthetic and perioperative management. We hope it will prove useful but we would emphasise that this, or any other book, is no substitute for experienced supervision, support and training.

- Is not a substitute for the major anaesthetic texts but concentrates on principles of management of the most challenging anaesthetic cases.

- Aims to provide guidance to help manage these patients in the perioperative period in line with modern concepts of critical care 'outreach' and the potential role of the anaesthetist as perioperative physician.

- Emphasises cardiovascular risk, cardiac disease and cardiac management as these are undoubtedly the most important aspects of perioperative anaesthetic risk.

- The choice of topics is, by nature of the size of text intended, selective but should appeal and be useful to the majority of practitioners. Important information not readily available in similar texts, e.g. a summary of all confidential enquiry into perioperative deaths (CEPOD) reports, perioperative renal failure, the role of the cardiology consult and indications for admission to high dependency unit (HDU) and intensive care unit (ICU) are included.

- The format is designed to provide easy access to information presented in a concise manner. We have tried to eliminate all superfluous material. Selected important or controversial references are presented as well as suggestions for Further reading. The style of the chapters vary. This is deliberate. Some relate more to basic principles, physiology, pharmacology, etc. – bookwork. Others are more practical in nature, discussing the principles of anaesthetic techniques for certain high-risk situations.

- The authors are all experienced practitioners working in a large, busy DGH with a high proportion of sick, elderly patients presenting for both elective and emergency surgery. The authors are committed to providing a high level of perioperative care of patients undergoing anaesthesia. We make no apologies for repetition of important principles and facts.

I McConachie
Blackpool
2001

CONTRIBUTORS

Blackpool Victoria Hospital, Whinney Heys Road, Blackpool FY3 8NR, England

Department of Anaesthesia
Dr A. Adams FRCS FRCA
Dr K. Paramesh FRCA
Dr C. Dunkley FRCA
Dr D.J. Counsell FRCA
Dr B. Lord FRCA
Dr D. Hume FRCA
Dr S. Vaughan MRCP FRCA
Dr M. Cutts MRCP FRCA
Dr S. Lakshmanan FRCA
Dr M. Hartley FRCA
Dr C. Harle FRCA
Dr G. Johnson FRCA
Dr M. Chamberlain FRCA
Dr A. Heard FRCA
Dr N. Harper FRCA
Dr V. Prasad FRCA
Dr J. Cupitt FRCA
Dr M. Bewsher FRCA
Dr I. McConachie FRCA

Department of Cardiology
Dr S. Bulugahapitiya MRCP
Dr D. Hesketh Roberts FRCP

Acute Pain Service
Ms F. Duncan SRN

1

EPIDEMIOLOGY AND IDENTIFICATION OF THE HIGH-RISK SURGICAL PATIENT

Patients that present for surgery may be at increased clinical risk for a variety of reasons. These reasons can be broadly divided into the following categories.

Availability of appropriately experienced staff

The confidential enquiry into peri-operative deaths (CEPOD) has identified the importance of training and adequate experience for medical staff. Training and, therefore, competence is an issue:

- 'Board-certified' trauma surgeons improve outcome following major trauma.[1]

- Trained specialists improve the outcome of septic shock in intensive care unit (ICU).[2]

Clinical volume for surgeons may be important:

- Studies have looked at both hospital volume and individual surgeons volume. Both may be important (with some evidence that 'high volume' hospital may compensate up to a point for 'low volume' surgeons).[3]

- Several studies have looked at bowel cancer surgery. There are significant differences in outcome between surgeons for colon cancer surgery. It has been suggested that such surgery should only be undertaken by specialist surgeons. One may assume that volume would be a factor in this and studies support this.

- However, one must be wary of uncritically accepting this – there are differences in surgical practice between the US and UK surgeons.

For example, in a paper showing importance of volume in colorectal surgery,[3] low volume was five or less cases in a *year*. High volume was > 10 cases a year (and these surgeons were in a minority). Few UK general surgeons would, therefore, not fall in the high volume group – with some performing that many in a month.

As regards, the anaesthetist, there have been few studies which have effectively come down to assessing the role of the *competence* of the anaesthetist on risk and outcome.

- One study of patients undergoing coronary artery surgery found that the only non–patient related factors influencing outcome were cardiac bypass time and the anaesthetist.[4]

One can expect more such studies in the future.

Timing of surgery

CEPOD has confirmed that surgery performed at night, when staff are more likely to be fatigued, is more hazardous and contributes to increased mortality.[5]

Availability of equipment

It is clear how the absence of basic equipment (e.g. capnography or pulse oximetry) might contribute to increased risk.

Patient factors

Many of these (see below) may be beyond the control or influence of the clinicians but may still be associated with increased risk or worse outcome.

Gender

The influence of gender on cardiovascular risk is discussed below. Some studies have investigated the role of gender in peri-operative risk and surgical risk and outcome:

- Females have significantly better outcomes including mortality and recurrence rates from melanomas.[6]

- The incidence of septic shock requiring intensive care is significantly less in females.[7] No differences in outcome, however, were demonstrated.

- Aligned with this is the observation that males have a higher incidence of infection following trauma.[8]

- Females have a worse outcome from IPPV but this was less important in predicting outcome than age, APACHE scores or presence of ARDS.[9]

- Females have a worse outcome following vascular surgery.[10]

Although gender may influence risks and outcome, this must be put into perspective and is only believed to be a minor risk factor overall. Vascular surgery may be an exception in that several studies suggest gender to be an important risk factor.

Age

Discussed as a cardiovascular risk factor below and also in the chapter on the elderly patient.

Race

The influence of a patient's race on risk and outcome is poorly understood and is a very sensitive issue – not least because of concerns that any such differences may reflect prejudice or access to health care. Differences in ethnic incidence and drug responses in hypertension have long been recognised. A few studies have examined race as a factor in surgical and peri-operative risk and outcome:

- Prostate cancer may be intrinsically more aggressive with a worse outcome in North American negroes.[11]

- There are similar results for endometrial cancer.[12]

Race has not been identified as an anaesthetic risk factor.

Genetic predisposition

The understanding of genetic predispositions to risk of sepsis and cardiac prognosis is still in its infancy. No work has been done on surgical outcomes but a genetic predisposition to high levels of angiotensin converting enzyme is associated with reduced survival following diagnosis of cardiac failure.[13] This may have implications for cardiac reserve and response to physiological stress peri-operatively. It is also very likely that the inflammatory response and response to infection is, in part, genetically predetermined.

Clinical conditions

There are numerous examples of high profile clinical conditions that readily predict high peri-operative risk:

- leaking abdominal aortic aneurysm,

- an unstarved patient with difficult intubation for emergency surgery,

- the emergency obstetric patient for caesarean section,

- fractured neck of femur,

- myopathic conditions,

- malignant hyperthermia,

- hereditary mastocystosis,

- latex allergy.

Many of these conditions are rare and would account for a small fraction of peri-operative deaths whilst others represent conditions that predispose to increased mortality for multifactorial reasons.

The majority of this chapter discusses cardiovascular disease as the most important factor in risk.

THE SIGNIFICANCE OF CARDIOVASCULAR DISEASE

There are currently two main theories as to how cardiac disease might contribute to peri-operative mortality in the surgical patient:

- **Myocardial ischaemia:** Tachycardia and increased myocardial oxygen demand increases shear stress on atherosclerotic plaques, which leads to plaque rupture, coronary thrombosis and myocardial infarction (MI).

- **Poor cardiopulmonary physiological reserve:** The physiological reserve of the heart and lungs is insufficient to meet the increased demands of surgery. In physiological terms, oxygen delivery does not fulfil oxygen consumption requirements. End-organ ischaemia results in multi-organ dysfunction syndrome (MODS) and death.

Interestingly, with respect to this second hypothesis, it has recently been shown that a pre-operative intramucosal gastric pH of < 7.35 predicted increased mortality.[14] pH$_i$ is a marker of blood supply to the stomach, and low values are thought to reflect inadequate oxygen delivery to the gut.

The second hypothesis also explains the importance of adequate pulmonary reserve and the contribution of pulmonary disease to surgical mortality in the peri-operative period. Pulmonary risk stratification is discussed in the next chapter.

RISK STRATIFICATION

The grading of patients into incremental levels of risk is known as risk stratification. There are a number of reasons why it is useful to identify who is at high risk:

- to identify those suitable for coronary revascularisation (either bypass grafting or angioplasty),

- to identify who would benefit from other peri-operative risk-reduction strategies.

Both strategies are likely to have major resource implications, however, the latter is increasingly being recognised as that most likely to improve outcome.[15]

CLINICAL FACTORS ASSOCIATED WITH INCREASED CARDIAC RISK

Advanced age (see also Chapter 7)

- Elderly patients have shorter life expectancy.

- Elderly patients have higher rates of treatment-related risks.

- Age increases the likelihood of coronary artery disease (CAD).

- The mortality of acute MI increases dramatically in the aged.

- Intra-operative or peri-operative MI has a higher mortality in the aged.

- CEPOD data shows for deaths within 30 days of surgery the peak age is 70–74 for males and 80–84 for females.

- In some elderly patients the risks of surgery may come close to risks of doing nothing.

Gender

- Premenopausal women have a lower incidence of CAD.

- CAD occurs 10 or more years later in women than in men.[16]

- Diabetic women have an increased risk, which is equivalent to men of the same age.

- The mortality rate following acute MI is greater for women than for men, but older age and diabetes mellitus account for much of this difference.[17]

Coronary artery disease

- A previous history of acute MI, bypass grafting, coronary angioplasty, or coronary angiography demonstrating coronary stenosis are all obvious indicators of ongoing CAD.

- Patients with a prior history of MI have an increased risk of peri-operative MI that is graded according to the time interval since their infarction (table 1.1).[18]

- The difficulty arises in identifying those patients with occult CAD.

Table 1.1 – Peri-operative infarction rates following a recent MI.[18]

Time since MI	Rate of new infarct (%)
> 6 months	5
Between 3 and 6 months	15
< 6 months	37

- In some patients symptoms may not occur due to functional limitation by arthritis or peripheral vascular disease.

It is these patients that may benefit from non-invasive testing to determine:

- the amount of myocardium critically perfused,

- the amount of stress required to produce ischaemia (ischaemic threshold),

- the ventricular function.

Non-invasive testing should not be performed in patients unsuitable for myocardial revascularisation.

- In those patients where the risk of coronary revascularisation is greater than the risk of non-cardiac surgery, the issue is whether to proceed with non-cardiac surgery anyway.

Hypertension

- Moderate hypertension is not an independent risk factor for peri-operative cardiovascular complications. There is thus, no need to delay surgery for mild or moderate hypertension with no associated metabolic or cardiovascular abnormalities.[19]

- However, as hypertension is associated with ischaemic heart disease, it should raise the index of suspicion.

- Poorly controlled hypertension can cause exaggerated intra-operative blood pressure variation and electrocardiograph (ECG) evidence of myocardial ischaemia, which has been shown to be a factor in post-operative cardiac morbidity.

- Effective pre-operative blood pressure control has been shown to reduce the incidence of peri-operative ischaemia so all antihypertensive medications should be continued during the peri-operative period.[17,20]

- Severe hypertension (diastolic > 110 mmHg) should be controlled before surgery when possible.

- Any decision to delay surgery for hypertension should balance the urgency of surgery against the potential benefit of aggressive medical optimisation.

- If urgent surgery is essential, intravenous β blockade can rapidly achieve effective control and reduce the number and duration of peri-operative coronary ischaemic episodes.

Congestive heart failure

- Congestive heart failure (CHF) has been identified in numerous studies as a predictor of a poor outcome in non-cardiac surgery.

- Validated predictive clinical signs include the presence of a third heart sound, and bibasal crackles.

- In Goldman's study,[21] the presence of a third heart sound or signs of CHF were associated with a substantially increased risk during non-cardiac surgery.

- Consideration of the aetiology of heart failure is particularly important; heart failure of ischaemic origin carries a greater significance and risk than that caused by hypertension.[19]

Valvular heart disease

With all murmurs one needs to determine:

- if the murmur is organic or simply a flow murmur,

- if the murmur is significant,

- whether endocarditis prophylaxis is required,

- the severity of the valvular lesion,

- if an echo is indicated.

Symptomatic stenotic lesions

- Symptomatic stenotic lesions are associated with severe peri-operative CHF or shock and normally require percutaneous valvotomy or valve replacement prior to surgery to reduce cardiac risk.

- Severe aortic stenosis poses the greatest risk and elective non-cardiac surgery should generally be postponed until fully assessed.[21]

- Mitral stenosis, although rare, increases the risk of CHF and balloon valvuloplasty or open repair may reduce peri-operative risk.[22]

- Mild or moderate stenosis requires careful avoidance of tachycardia to minimise the reduction in diastolic filling time that can precipitate severe pulmonary congestion.

Symptomatic regurgitant valve disease

- Symptomatic regurgitant valve disease is usually better tolerated peri-operatively and may be stabilised pre-operatively with intensive medical therapy and monitoring.

- Usually treated definitively with valve repair or replacement either after or at the same time as non-cardiac surgery if left ventricular (LV) function is adequate.

- Aortic regurgitation requires attention to volume control and afterload reduction.

- In severe aortic regurgitation slow heart rates increase the volume of regurgitation by increasing the amount of time in diastole.

- Moderate tachycardia is preferred as faster heart rates reduce diastole and, therefore, reduces the time for regurgitation.

Arrhythmias and conduction abnormalities

- Although both supraventricular and ventricular arrhythmias have been identified as independent risk factors for coronary events in the peri-operative period,[21] they are probably significant because they reflect the presence of underlying serious cardiopulmonary disease, drug toxicity, or metabolic abnormality.

Diabetes mellitus

- Diabetes mellitus increases both the likelihood and extent of CAD.

- Myocardial ischaemia and MI are more likely to be silent with diabetes mellitus.[23]

Peripheral vascular disease and cerebrovascular disease

- These conditions confer an increased risk for cardiac complications, since many of the risk factors contributing to peripheral vascular disease (diabetes mellitus, smoking, hyperlipidemia) are also risk factors for CAD.

- As mentioned above, symptoms suggestive of CAD may be masked by exercise limitations.

- The presence of peripheral vascular disease is more important as a predictor of cardiac events than the actual vascular operation to be performed.[19]

SCORING SYSTEMS

Scoring systems are usually derived from the statistical analysis of large population groups where certain factors predictive of increased risk are identified and weighted according to their individual significance.

The ideal scoring system for predicting clinical risk would be:

- simple to use,
- highly sensitive,
- highly specific,
- high positive predictive value,
- cheap without requiring use of expensive resources or tests.

There are numerous scoring systems that have been published over the years, the most important of these include:

- American Society of Anesthesiologists 'ASA' Status,[24]
- Goldman's Cardiac Risk Index,[21]
- Detsky's Modified Cardiac Risk Index,[25]
- Lee's Revised Cardiac Risk Index.[26]

American Society of Anesthesiologists 'ASA' Status

This classification of physical status was originally introduced in 1941 with seven classes, but was revised to its final form of just five classes in 1963[24] (table 1.2). The main points to note regarding ASA status include:

- it stratifies patients by simple assessment of physical status,
- no expensive tests or clinical resources required,
- there can be considerable observer variability of patients' physical status.

Important factors not taken into account include:

- age – some workers add an extra grade on for age >75 years,
- complexity of operation,
- duration of operation,
- whether the disease process is incidental or factorial in current illness.

Table 1.2 – American Association of Anesthesiologists 'ASA' Status and mortality ranges for each class.[24]

ASA class	Definition	Mortality (%)
I	Healthy	0–0.3
II	Mild systemic disease with no functional limitation	0.3–1.4
III	Severe systemic disease with functional limitation	1.8–5.4
IV	Severe systemic disease – constant threat to life	7.8–25.9
V	Moribund patient unlikely to survive 24 h with or without operation	9.4–57.8
E	Suffix added to denote emergency operation	

Wolters et al.[27] recently investigated whether the ASA classification and the presence of peri-operative risk factors could be used as a predictive tool either for outcome or post-operative complications; factors shown to correlate with increasing class of ASA included:

- intra-operative blood loss,
- duration of operation,
- duration of post-operative ventilation,
- post-operative wound and urinary tract infections,
- length of ICU stay and hospital stay,
- rates of pulmonary and cardiac complications,
- in-hospital mortality.

The variables found to be most important for predicting complications were a high ASA class, having a major operation, and having an emergency operation.

Many retrospective studies and a couple of prospective studies have demonstrated a correlation between ASA and peri-operative mortality and justifies the use of ASA classification as a crude predictor of patient outcome.

Goldman's Cardiac Risk Index

This landmark paper was published in the NEJM 1977,[21] and is a well-known method for stratifying risk (table 1.3).

Its limitations are few but include:

- The index overestimated the incidence of cardiac morbidity in Class IV patients undergoing non-cardiac surgery.
- The index underestimated risk in Class I and II patients undergoing aortic surgery.
- The study group included elective non-emergent cases only.

Table 1.3 – Goldman's Cardiac Risk Index.[21]

Criteria		Points
History	Age > 70	5
	MI in previous 6 months	10
Examination	S_3 gallop or jugular venous distension	11
	Important valvular aortic stenosis	3
ECG	Rhythm other than sinus or PACs	7
	> 5 PVCs/min at any time before operation	7
General status	$pO_2 < 60$ or $pCO_2 > 50$ mmHg	3
	$K < 3.0$ or $HCO_3 < 20$ mmol/l	
	Urea > 18 mmol/l or Cr $> 240\ \mu$mol	
	Abnormal AST (SGOT)	
	Signs of chronic liver disease	
	Patient bedridden from non-cardiac causes	
Operation	Intraperitoneal, intrathoracic, or aortic	3
	emergency	4
Total possible points		53

Group	Score	Life-threatening complications (%)	Deaths (%)
I	0–5	0.7	0.2
II	6–12	5	1.5
III	13–25	11	2.3
IV	26–53	22	56

Subsequently a number of authors attempted to improve upon the original Goldman's Cardiac Risk Index. In 1986 Detsky *et al.*, published the Modified Cardiac Risk Index[25] in which a number of other clinical conditions were incorporated:

- Canadian cardiovascular society angina Classes III and IV,

- unstable angina,

- history of pulmonary oedema.

Since then other authors have suggested the addition of coronary perfusion scans or dobutamine stress echocardiography as a means of improving sensitivity and specificity.

Revised Cardiac Risk Index

The Revised Cardiac Risk Index (table 1.4) is the most recent scoring systems and was introduced by Lee *et al.* in 1999.[26] The index was derived from a population of 4000 patients, and identified the risk of major cardiac complications in a population undergoing major non-emergent non-cardiac surgery.

Table 1.4 – Revised Cardiac Risk Index.[26]

Risk factors	Inclusion criteria
Ischaemic heart disease	MI
	Q waves
	Angina
	Nitrates
	Positive exercise stress test
CHF	History
	Examination
	CXR
Cerebrovascular disease	Stroke
	TIA
Insulin treated diabetes	
Creatinine	$> 177 \mu$mol
High-risk surgery	AAA repair
	Thoracic
	Abdominal

Revised Cardiac Risk Index	No. of factors	Proportion of population (%)	Major cardiac complications (%)
Class I	0	36	0.4
Class II	1	39	1.1
Class III	2	18	4.6
Class IV	3 or more	7	9.7

Patients with 0 or one risk factor accounted for 75% of population and had a risk of major cardiac event of 1.5%.
Patients with two risk factors accounted for 18% of the population group with a risk of major cardiac event of 4.6%.
Patients with three or more risk factors accounted for 7% of the population group with a risk of major cardiac event of 9.7%.

Major cardiac complications included MI, pulmonary oedema, ventricular fibrillation or primary cardiac arrest, or complete heart block.

Its advantages over the earlier scoring systems include:

- only six prognostic factors,

- simple variables,

- dependent on presence or absence of conditions rather than estimating disease severity,

- less reliance on clinical assessment and judgement,

- could easily be incorporated on pre-operative evaluation forms.

The shortcomings of the system are that:

- it is not applicable to emergency surgery,

- it is not applicable to lower-risk populations,

- it may not be as reliable for pre-selected high-risk populations such as patients undergoing major vascular surgery.

APACHE systems

APACHE is an acronym for **A**cute **P**hysiology and **C**hronic **H**ealth **E**valuation. APACHE II and III are scoring systems in widespread use in ICUs, but are unsuitable as a pre-operative risk stratification tools because for score generation requires 12 physiological parameters from the first 24 h of care as well as age and previous health status.

Possum

Possum is an acronym for the **P**hysiological and **O**perative **S**everity **S**core for the **E**numeration of Mortality and **M**orbidity. Copeland *et al.*[28] developed this scoring system in 1991 for audit purposes. It requires 12 physiological variables, a number of operative severity score factors and is reliant on outcome for final score and, therefore, is not suitable for pre-operative risk prediction:

- It has mainly been utilised in the UK to date.

- Its main use is to compare hospitals for audit purposes and identify differences between individual surgeons.

- The score may overpredict mortality in low-risk patients.

- It does not predict mortality accurately for ruptured aortic aneurysms.[29]

- Possum is better than APACHE II in predicting mortality in high dependency unit (HDU) patients.[30]

- For colorectal surgery, predicted mortality with Possum equals actual mortality.[31]

AMERICAN COLLEGE OF CARDIOLOGISTS/AMERICAN HEART ASSOCIATION GUIDELINES

In 1996 the American College of Cardiologists and the American Heart Association (ACC/AHA) introduced guidelines for the peri-operative cardiovascular evaluation of patients undergoing non-cardiac surgery.[19]

- The guidelines reflected the failings of the scoring systems and were designed to provide central, evidenced-based advice as a strategy to reduce litigation claims for suboptimal pre-operative management in the US.

- They were also an attempt to rationalise the increasing demand for expensive risk stratification tests being requested as part of routine pre-operative assessments.

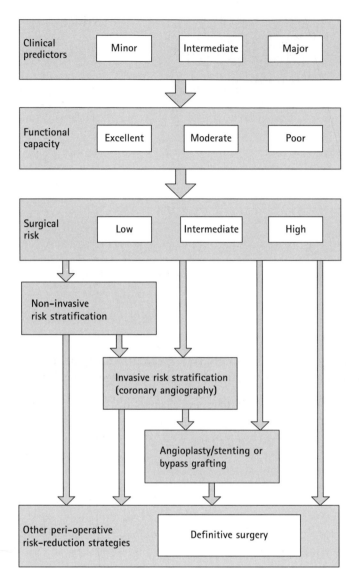

Figure 1.1 – Illustration of stepwise process to aid clinical risk assessment and stratification.[19]

The guidelines proposed a sequential stepwise strategy of risk assessment based upon (figure 1.1):

- the identification of certain clinical predictors of risk,
- an assessment of the patients functional capacity,
- the type of surgery to be undertaken.

Table 1.5 – ACC AHA clinical predictors of coronary risk.[19]

Minor clinical predictors	Intermediate predictors	Major predictors
Advanced age	Mild stable angina Class I/II	Unstable coronary syndromes
Abnormal ECG	Previous MI by Hx or Q waves	Recent MI < 30 days
LVH	Compensated CCF	Unstable or severe angina
LBBB	IDDM	Decompensated CCF
ST-T abnormalities		Significant arrhythmias
Absence of sinus rhythm		High grade AV block
Low functional capacity		Symptomatic ventricular
Previous CVA		arrhythmias
Uncontrolled hypertension		Supraventricular tachyarrhythmias
		Severe valvular heart disease

Clinical predictors of coronary risk

Table 1.5 lists a number of clinical predictors of increasing risk for MI, CHF, and death established by several authors based on multivariate analysis:[19]

- Patients with **minor predictors** do not usually require any further non-invasive testing.

- Patients possessing **intermediate predictors** may be further stratified according to their functional capacity and surgery-specific risk.

- **Major clinical predictors** are so predictive of high risk that further stratification, using functional capacity and surgery-specific risk, is usually unnecessary. These patients invariably require further non-invasive risk stratification testing, and this often results in the delay or cancellation of all but emergency surgery.

Interestingly, the guidelines class a history of MI or pathological Q waves by ECG as an intermediate predictor, whereas a recent MI is a major predictor. They admit that there are no adequate clinical trials on which to base firm recommendations, but suggest a delay of 4–6 weeks after MI before anaesthetising for elective surgery.

Functional capacity

- Assessment of an individual's capacity to perform a number of different physical tasks has been shown to correlate with maximum oxygen uptake (vO_2 max) by treadmill testing.

- Exercise tolerance or physical fitness can be assessed in metabolic equivalent levels, or 'METs', which is a validated method of determining functional capacity from the patients history (table 1.6).

Table 1.6 – Metabolic equivalent levels with examples of common daily tasks.[32]

Metabolic levels	Equivalent activity
1 MET	Eat
	Dress
	Use toilet
	Walk indoors around house
	Light house-work
	Walk on level ground at 2–3 mph
4 METs	Climb flight of stairs
	Walk up hill
	Run a short distance
	Heavy house-work, scrubbing floors, moving heavy furniture
	Walk on level ground at 4 mph
	Recreational activity: golf, bowling, dancing, tennis
10 METs	Strenuous sports: swimming, football, skiing, basketball

- Peri-operative and long-term cardiac risk is increased in patients unable to achieve four 'MET' levels of exercise during normal day-to-day living.[32]

- Poor functional capacity in patients with chronic CAD or in those convalescing after an acute cardiac event is associated with an increased risk of subsequent cardiac morbidity and mortality.

- Decreased functional capacity may be a result of several factors, including inadequate cardiac reserve, advanced age, transient myocardial dysfunction from myocardial ischaemia, deconditioning, and poor pulmonary reserve.

Surgical risk

In elective surgery the magnitude of cardiac risk has been stratified to the magnitude of the surgical procedure and to major thoracic, abdominal, or vascular surgery, especially in patients of 70 years or older.[19]

In the ACC/AHA guidelines, surgical procedures are classified as low, intermediate, or high risk (table 1.7) and are based upon the likelihood of non-fatal MI or death from cardiac causes:

- Low-risk procedures are usually short, with minimal fluid shifts, while higher-risk operations tend to be prolonged with large fluid shifts and greater potential for post-operative myocardial ischaemia and respiratory depression.

- Not surprisingly, major vascular procedures represent the highest-risk procedures.

Table 1.7 – Grade of risk (with reported cardiac risk) with type of surgical procedure. Risk is for combined incidence of cardiac death and non-fatal MI.[19]

Low risk (<1%)	Intermediate risk (<5%)	High risk (>5%)
Endoscopic procedures	Carotid endarterectomy	Emergent major (particularly elderly)
Superficial procedures	Head and neck	Aortic and other major vascular surgery
Cataract surgery	Intraperitoneal and intrathoracic	Peripheral vascular
Breast surgery	Orthopaedic	Anticipated prolonged surgical procedures
	Prostate	Associated with large fluid shifts/blood loss

- Superficial and ophthalmologic procedures represent the lowest risk and are rarely associated with excess morbidity and mortality.

- In the intermediate-risk category, morbidity and mortality vary, depending on the surgical location and extent of the procedure.

- Emergency surgery is a special case as the necessity for immediate surgery precludes the time needed to fully evaluate and optimise these patients. The result is that cardiac complications are two to five times more likely to occur with emergency surgical procedures.[33] For example, in asymptomatic elective abdominal aortic aneurysms repair, the mortality rate is 3.5% but this rises to 42% if ruptured.[34]

Individual clinician-based patient assessment

- This is a clinical philosophy that is gaining increasing acceptance as a valid alternative to the use of rigid risk scoring systems and guidelines.

- It relies on the history, physical examination and acquired clinical experience to identify potential markers of increased risk.

- The difference between this approach and the use of scoring systems is that clinicians have a unique ability to integrate the numerous other factors surrounding the patients' presentation for surgery that contribute to peri-operative risk but would be impossible to quantify and validate in a scoring system.

- The result is a clinician-based assessment of risk that is specifically tailored to each individual patient. Diagnostic testing and risk-reduction strategies are then **selectively** instigated, according to this experience, where clinical and financial resources permit.

- Clinician-based judgement strategies are thus adaptable to individual clinical situations rather than rigidly applying an index score alone when estimating peri-operative risk.

- This philosophy maintains that risk scoring systems and guidelines are most useful, therefore, only as guides for inexperienced clinicians.

Non-invasive tests to stratify cardiovascular risk

The purpose of supplemental pre-operative testing is:

- to identify the presence of important pre-operative myocardial ischaemia or cardiac arrhythmias,
- to estimate peri-operative cardiac risk and long-term prognosis,
- **and** to provide an objective measure of **functional capacity**.

They should not be performed if they are unlikely to influence management.

The ideal test for stratification should be:

- simple,
- cheap,
- non-invasive,
- sensitive,
- specific,
- capable of identifying who will be at risk for peri-operative cardiac events,
- capable of identifying those patients with correctable coronary lesions.

Risk stratification tests should be restricted to patients clinically assessed as high risk (and occasionally significant intermediate risk) because:

- limiting their use in this way has been shown to enhance predictive accuracy,
- uncontrolled use would have significant resource and cost implications.

A classification of non-invasive risk stratification tests is offered in table 1.8.

Ambulatory electrocardiographic monitoring

This involves making a 24- to 48-h pre-operative ambulatory ECG record. Episodes of ischaemia may be predictive of early and late ischaemic cardiac events.

However, there are a number of limitations:

- It cannot be performed in a significant percentage of patients with baseline ECG changes as it is less predictive in high-risk groups with abnormal ECGs.

Table 1.8 – Non-invasive tests currently available to stratify cardiovascular risk.

Modality	Rest tests	'Stress' tests

ECG	Resting ECG	Ambulatory ECG
		Stress ECG with exercise
		Stress ECG with inotropes
		  Dobutamine
		  Arbutamine

Myocardial nuclear imaging	Myocardial rest perfusion imaging	Myocardial stress perfusion in
		  Coronary vasodilators
		    Adenosine
		    Dipyridamole
		  Inotropes
		    Dobutamine
		    Arbutamine

	Radionuclide ventriculography	

Echocardiography	Resting echo	Inotrope stress echo
		  Dobutamine
		  Arbutamine

Invasive/exercise	vO_2 max Coronary angiography	

- The test only provides a binary outcome (normal/abnormal) and, therefore, cannot further stratify the high-risk group in order to identify the subset for which coronary angiography should be considered.

Ambulatory ECG should, therefore, be restricted to identifying patients for whom additional surveillance or intervention might be beneficial. It should not be used as the only diagnostic test to identify patients for coronary angiography.

'Stress' testing

- In both animal and human models a coronary stenosis will only start to produce flow limitation at rest when the cross sectional diameter is reduced by 85–90%.

- Under conditions of maximal flow, however, stenoses with as little as 45% reduction in cross sectional diameter will cause flow limitation.

- Clinically this phenomenon manifests as effort-induced angina.

- Thus the sensitivity of diagnostic physiological tests are markedly improved with increased flow enabling the detection of lesser stenoses.

Increasing coronary blood flow can be achieved in a number of ways including graded exercise, pacing and pharmacological agents, and these methods are combined with various methods of detecting ischaemia including ECG, echocardiography and nuclear myocardial imaging.

Exercise stress testing

Exercise is most commonly employed in exercise ECGs under the Bruce Protocol.

Although not validated for improving outcome, it is extremely useful as a predictor of pre-operative risk as it identifies patients with **both poor functional capacity and associated ischaemia.**[19]

It is effective at stratifying coronary risk according to:

- degree of functional incapacity,
- ischaemic symptoms,
- ischaemic severity (stage of onset, depth and duration of ST segment depression),
- haemodynamic instability,
- electrical instability.

The degree of positivity of test correlates with extent and severity of disease.

The risk of peri-operative cardiac events and long-term risk is significantly increased in patients with an abnormal exercise ECG at low workloads.

The sensitivity gradient for detecting obstructive coronary disease is dependent on:

- severity of stenosis,
- criteria used for a positive test,
- extent of disease, i.e. the presence of a prior clinical history.

For example, in patients with no cardiac history and a normal resting ECG, only 20–25% of patients will have an abnormal exercise ECG, whereas in patients with a prior history of MI or an abnormal rest ECG 35–50% of patients will have an abnormal exercise ECG. However, it should be borne in mind that:

- As many as 50% of patients with significant CAD and adequate levels of exercise can still produce a normal exercise ECG.[35]
- There is no evidence to support its use in low-risk groups.

Pharmacological stressors

Inotropes

- Commonly used inotropes include dobutamine and the newer agent arbutamine. These drugs increase myocardial oxygen demand through inotropic stimulation.

- They can often achieve coronary blood flows greater than with exercise but not as great as with adenosine or dipyridamole.

- They tend to be used in patients with asthma who cannot tolerate vasodilators.

- Dobutamine is best avoided in patients with serious arrhythmias and severe hypertension or hypotension.

Coronary vasodilators

These agents produce non-physiological and sometimes supra-physiological increases in coronary flow without altering the metabolic demands of the heart.

- **Adenosine** is a breakdown product of ATP metabolism and is a potent coronary vasodilator. In conditions of oxygen starvation rising adenosine levels result in coronary vasodilation linking coronary blood flow to myocardial oxygen demand.

- **Dipyridamole** inhibits the breakdown of free adenosine causing levels to rise and thereby produces coronary vasodilatation as described above.

- **Methylxanthines** (e.g. caffeine) are competitive inhibitors of adenosine at purinergic receptors and patients are advised to avoid these for at least 6–8 h prior to testing achieve maximal coronary vasodilator effect.

All these agents can induce or exacerbate bronchospasm, and their use is relatively contraindicated in asthmatics. Unexpected severe bronchospasm can be readily antagonised with intravenous aminophylline. Dipyridamole should also be avoided in patients with critical carotid disease. Other adverse effects include headaches, flushing and hypotension.

Examples of some non-invasive tests that employ pharmacological stressors include:

Dobutamine stress echocardiography

- Provides an opportunity to assess both LV and valvular function.

- Can be performed safely and with acceptable patient tolerance.

- Very accurate in identifying patients with significant angiographic coronary disease.

- The published experience of dobutamine stress echocardiography to assess peri-operative risk before vascular and non-vascular surgery is relatively small compared with the published literature on exercise testing or intravenous dipyridamole myocardial perfusion imaging.

- Adding atropine to those patients who fail to meet the target heart rate improves sensitivity.

- Several studies suggest that the degree of wall motion abnormalities and/or wall motion change at low infusion rates of dobutamine is especially important.

Myocardial perfusion stress imaging

- Myocardial uptake of perfusion agents is dependent on blood flow rather than oxygen demand or metabolic activity.

- Resting images alone can be done but sensitivity is very low and is significantly increased if stress images are taken.

- Any of the agents described above can be used to increase coronary blood flow with the most data available for dipyridamole.

- The tests have high sensitivity and specificity for peri-operative coronary events.

The technique involves the injection of a radionuclide during peak blood flow. The main isotopes in use are:

- **Thallium-201** is a monovalent cation and like potassium is taken into myocardial cells by Na–K ATPase. It emits both X-rays and gamma radiation and has a relatively long half-life of 73.1 h. It readily and rapidly redistributes with myocardial blood flow so that a 2nd dose is not required to obtain rest images. The main disadvantage with thallium is the low energy of its emitted radiation resulting in significant soft tissue attenuation, which can affect image quality and hinder image interpretation.

- **Technetium-99m** is an isotope with many advantages over thallium for producing better quality myocardial images; it emits radiation at a higher energy resulting in less attenuation, and its shorter half-life of 6 h allows larger doses. Technetium-99m does not redistribute and, therefore, requires separate stress and rest injections. The main compound incorporating this isotope is known as Sestamibi. Unfortunately the superior image quality of images produced with Technetium-99m has yet to be shown to improve diagnostic accuracy.

Images of the myocardium are then compared at peak or stress coronary flow and after a delay, at rest. Exercise-induced ischaemia results in a perfusion defect on the stress images that fills in or redistributes on the rest images. MI manifests as fixed perfusion defects on both the stress and rest images.

Severe myocardial disease causing exercise-induced pump failure can also be detected using this technique. The LV decompensates with a fall in stroke volume and ejection fraction with a resultant increase in LV end diastolic pressure and diameter; on the stress images the ventricular cavity is larger and the ventricle wall is thinner. As a further consequence of the rise in LV end diastolic pressure, raised levels of isotope will often accumulate in the lungs.

Subendocardial ischaemia results in reduced endocardial uptake of isotope and may also appear as LV dilatation.

In increasing grade of risk, possible scan results are:

Normal scan < fixed defects < redistribution defects

Furthermore, as the size of the defect increases, risk significantly increases.

Digital quantitation of scan abnormalities improves positive predictive value and is improving alongside advances in technology.

The need for caution in routine screening with a dipyridamole–thallium stress test of all patients before vascular surgery was raised by Baron *et al.*[36] In this review of 457 patients undergoing elective abdominal aortic surgery, the presence of definite CAD on clinical assessment and age > 65 years were better predictors of cardiac complications than perfusion imaging.

LV ejection fraction

Resting ventricular function (including LV ejection fraction) is usually determined by echocardiography but may also be determined by radionuclide angiography, gated radionuclide imaging or contrast ventriculography.

Ejection fraction determined by echo is limited in accuracy as the formula used in its calculation assumes the ventricle to be a sphere and the diameters of the 'full sphere' and 'empty sphere' are only measured in one plane.

Increased risks of complications are associated with:

- LV ejection fraction < 35%,[19]

- diastolic and systolic dysfunction are markers for post-operative congestive cardiac failure, and in critically ill patients, death.

It is important to note that resting LV function is not a *consistent* predictor of perioperative ischaemic events.

Recommendations for non-invasive testing[19]

In most ambulatory patients, the test of choice is exercise ECG testing, which can both provide an estimate of functional capacity and detect myocardial ischaemia through changes in the ECG and haemodynamic response.

In patients with contraindications to exercise ECG testing, e.g. left bundle branch block or LV hypertrophy, other techniques may be preferable such as:

- exercise echocardiography,

- exercise myocardial perfusion imaging.

In those patients unable to perform adequate exercise the following may be more useful:

- dipyridamole–thallium scanning;

- dobutamine echocardiography;

- finally if there is an additional question about valvular dysfunction, the echocardiographic stress test is favoured;

- in many instances, either myocardial stress perfusion imaging or stress echocardiography are appropriate.

In a recent meta-analysis assessing the use of, ambulatory ECG, dobutamine stress echocardiography, radionuclide ventriculography and dipyridamole–thallium scanning, for predicting adverse cardiac outcome after vascular surgery, all tests had a similar predictive value, with overlapping confidence intervals.

Other important points to note include:

- Local expertise and experience of a test is probably more important than the particular type of test.

- Selective rather than routine testing improves cost effectiveness.

- Non-selective blanket tests are not cost effective and are an inefficient use of resources because at the extremes of risk these tests add very little predictive value.

Invasive testing (coronary angiography)

For very high-risk patients it may be sometimes more appropriate to proceed with coronary angiography rather than perform a non-invasive test. These might include:

- patients with major clinical predictors,

- advanced ischaemic risk such as unstable angina or residual ischaemia following a recent MI.

In addition it may be reasonable to consider coronary angiography and percutaneous transluminal coronary angioplasty (PTCA) or coronary artery bypass grafting (CABG) before non-cardiac surgery when the stress of elective non-cardiac surgery is likely to exceed the stress of daily life.

However, before proceeding to coronary angiography one needs to ascertain that the patient is fit enough for either PTCA or CABG. If not angiography only adds to the cost and will not improve outcome.

- As far as the new treatment modality of PTCA is concerned, there is little evidence available at present concerning its pre-operative use to optimise patients for non-cardiac surgery.

- Indeed there are no controlled trials comparing peri-operative cardiac outcome after PTCA versus medical therapy.

- A number of small observational series have suggested that cardiac death is infrequent in patients who have coronary angioplasty before non-cardiac surgery.

- Observational studies have shown a risk reduction for non-cardiac surgery after coronary bypass.

PRE-OPERATIVE ASSESSMENT AND RISK

The aim of pre-operative assessment is to minimise morbidity and mortality.

Three questions should be asked when assessing surgical patients with the aim of minimising operative risk:

1. Is the patient's medical and physiological status optimum?

2. If not, can the patient's status be improved (time permitting)?

3. If not, should the operation still proceed? In other words do the risks of not operating outweigh the risks of operating. For example, medical status is almost irrelevant if the operation is clearly life saving. Thus, no patient is 'not fit' for surgery – it just depends on the urgency of the situation.

Pre-operative assessment should identify those patients who are at high risk of pre- or post-operative organ failures. Such patients may need additional monitoring and may warrant admission to ICU or an HDU post-operatively for organ function monitoring or support.

Once the risk has been established and attempts have been made to optimise the patient's condition (i.e. reduce the risk), patients and their families may need to decide whether to proceed with surgery. One of the responsibilities of the anaesthetist is be able to give the patient relevant and accurate information on risk in order to help them decide. Unfortunately few patients will have read the chapter in this text on the meaning of risk!

Further reading

Adams AM, Smith AF. Risk perception and communication: recent developments and implications for anaesthesia. *Anaesthesia* 2001; **56**: 745–55.

References

1. Rogers FB, Simons R, Hoyt DB *et al*. In-house board-certified surgeons improve outcome for severely injured patients: a comparison of two university centers. *J Trauma* 1993; **34**: 871–5.

2. Reynolds HN, Haupt MT, Thill-Baharozian MC *et al*. Impact of critical care physician staffing on patients with septic shock in a university hospital medical intensive care unit. *JAMA* 1988; **260**: 3446–50.

3. Harmon JW, Tang DG, Gordon TA *et al*. Hospital volume can serve as a surrogate for surgeon volume for achieving excellent outcomes in colorectal resection. *Ann Surg* 1999; **230**: 404–11.

4. Merry AF, Ramage MC, Whitlock RM *et al*. First-time coronary artery bypass grafting: the anaesthetist as a risk factor. *Br J Anaesth* 1992; **68**: 6–12.

5. Campling EA, Devlin HB, Hoile RW *et al*. Who operates when. *The report of the National Confidential Enquiry into Perioperative Deaths 1996/1997*. NCEPOD, London, 1997.

6. Stidham KR, Johnson JL, Seigler HF. Survival superiority of females with melanoma. A multivariate analysis of 6383 patients exploring the significance of gender in prognostic outcome. *Arch Surg* 1994; **129**: 316–24.

7. Wichmann MW, Inthorn D, Andress HJ *et al*. Incidence and mortality of severe sepsis in surgical intensive care patients: the influence of patient gender on disease process and outcome. *Int Care Med* 2000; **26**: 167–72.

8. Offner PJ, Moore EE, Biffl WL. Male gender is a risk factor for major infections after surgery. *Arch Surg* 1999; **134**: 935–8.

9. Kollef MH, O'Brien JD, Silver P. The impact of gender on outcome from mechanical ventilation. *Chest* 1997; **111**: 434–41.

10. Norman PE, Semmens JB, Lawrence-Brown M *et al*. The influence of gender on outcome following peripheral vascular surgery: a review. *Cardiovasc Surg* 2000; **8**: 111–15.

11. Moul JW, Douglas TH, McCarthy WF *et al*. Black race is an adverse prognostic factor for prostate cancer recurrence following radical prostatectomy in an equal access health care setting. *J Urol* 1996; **155**: 1667–73.

12. Connell PP, Rotmensch J, Waggoner SE *et al.* Race and clinical outcome in endometrial carcinoma. *Obstet Gynecol* 1999; **94**: 713–20.

13. Andersson B, Sylven C. The DD genotype of the angiotensin-converting enzyme gene is associated with increased mortality in idiopathic heart failure. *J Am Coll Cardiol* 1996; **28**: 162–7.

14. Poeze M, Takala J, Greve JWM, Ramsay G. Pre-operative tonometry is predictive for mortality and morbidity in high-risk surgical patients. *Int Care Med* 2000; **26**: 1272–81.

15. Kelion AD, Banning AP. Is simple clinical assessment adequate for cardiac risk stratification before elective non-cardiac surgery. *Lancet* 1999; **354**: 1838.

16. Castelli WP. Epidemiology of coronary heart disease: the Framingham study. *Am J Med* 1984; **76**: 4–12.

17. Becker RC, Terrin M, Ross R *et al.* and the Thrombolysis in Myocardial Infarction Investigators. Comparison of clinical outcomes for women and men after acute myocardial infarction. *Ann Intern Med* 1994; **120**: 638–45.

18. Shah KB, Kleinman BS, Rao TLK *et al.* Angina and other risk factors in patients with cardiac diseases undergoing non-cardiac operations. *Anesth Analg* 1990; **70**: 240–7.

19. Eagle KA, Brundage BH, Chaitman BR *et al.* Guidelines for perioperative cardiovascular evaluation for non-cardiac surgery: an abridged version of the report of the American College of Cardiology/American Heart Association Task Force on Practice Guidelines. *J Am Coll Cardiol* 1996; **27**: 910–48.

20. Goldman L, Caldera DL. Risks of general anesthesia and elective operation in the hypertensive patient. *Anesthesiology* 1979; **50**: 285–92.

21. Goldman L, Caldera DL, Nussbaum SR *et al.* Multifactorial index of cardiac risk in non-cardiac surgical procedures. *N Engl J Med* 1977; **297**: 845–50.

22. Reyes VP, Raju BS, Wynne J, Stephenson *et al.* Percutaneous balloon valvuloplasty compared with open surgical commissurotomy for mitral stenosis. *N Engl J Med* 1994; **331**: 961–96.

23. Alpert JS, Chipkin SR, Aronin N. Diabetes mellitus and silent myocardial ischemia. *Adv Cardiol* 1990; **37**: 279–303.

24. ASA. New classification of physical status. *Anaesthesiology* 1963; **24**: 111.

25. Detsky AS, Abrams HB, Forbath N, Scott JG, Hillard JR. Cardiac assessment for patients undergoing non-cardiac surgery. A multifactorial clinical risk index. *Arch Int Med* 1986; **146**: 2131–4.

26. Lee TH, Marcantonio ER, Mangione CM *et al.* Derivation and prospective validation of a simple index for prediction of cardiac risk of major non-cardiac surgery. *Circulation* 1999; **100**: 1043–9.

27. Wolters U, Wolf T, Stutzer H, Schroder T. ASA classification and peri-operative variables as predictors of postoperative outcome. *Br J Anaes* 1996; **77**: 217–22.

28. Copeland GP, Jones D, Waiters M. POSSUM: a scoring system for surgical audit. *Br J Surg* 1991; **78**: 355–60.

29. Lazarides MK, Arvanitis DP, Drista H *et al.* POSSUM and APACHE II scores do not predict the outcome of ruptured infrarenal aortic aneurysms. *Ann Vasc Surg* 1997; **11**: 155–8.

30. Jones DR, Copeland GP, de Cossart L. Comparison of POSSUM with APACHE II for prediction of outcome from a surgical high-dependency unit. *Br J Surg* 1992; **79**: 1293–6.

31. Sagar PM, Hartley MN, Mancey-Jones B *et al.* Comparative audit of colorec-tal resection with the POSSUM scoring system. *Br J Surg* 1994; **81**: 1492–4.

32. Hlatky MA, Boineau RE, Higginbotham MB, Lee KL, Mark DB, Califf RM, Cobb FR, Pryor DB. A brief self-administered questionnaire to determine functional capacity (the Duke Activity Status Index). *Am J Cardiol* 1989; **64**: 651–4.

33. Mangano DT. Perioperative cardiac morbidity. *Anesthesiology* 1990; **72**: 153–84.

34. Taylor LM Jr, Porter JM. Basic data related to clinical decision-making in abdominal aortic aneurysms. *Ann Vasc Surg* 1987; **1**: 502–4.

35. Chaitman BR. The changing role of the exercise electrocardiogram as a diag-nostic and prognostic test for chronic ischemic heart disease. *J Am Coll Cardiol* 1986; **8**: 1195–210.

36. Baron JF, Mundler O, Bertrand M, Vicaut E, Barre E, Godet G, Samama CM *et al.* Dipyridamole–thallium scintigraphy and gated radionuclide angiography to assess cardiac risk before abdominal aortic surgery. *N Engl J Med* 1994; **330**: 663–9.

2

RESPIRATORY RISK AND COMPLICATIONS

There is now an increasing volume of literature regarding the identification of the patient at risk of respiratory complications:

- Respiratory complications are at least as, and sometimes more common than cardiac complications.[1]

However, reaching a consensus on what constitutes a postoperative respiratory complication has proved difficult in recent years and has significantly hindered research in this area. Improvements in the health of the population, advances in anaesthesia and surgery and reduction in prevalence of smoking amongst the population have all combined to cause problems interpreting the significance of some of the early studies on respiratory risk and complications.

It is now increasingly gaining acceptance that significant respiratory complications are those that affect outcome. These are problems that prolong hospital or intensive care unit (ICU) stay, or alternatively contribute to morbidity or mortality.[2–4] They include:

- pneumonia,

- respiratory failure requiring mechanical ventilation,

- bronchospasm,

- atelectasis,

- exacerbation of chronic underlying disease.

Factors that have been shown to be predictive of postoperative pulmonary respiratory complications can be subdivided into patient- and surgery-related risk factors.

PATIENT-RELATED FACTORS

The relative increases in risk associated with the presence of patient-related factors is given in table 2.1.

Smoking

Smoking has long been recognised as a respiratory risk factor for patients both with and without chronic lung disease, and causes a 3–4-fold increase in the incidence of pulmonary complications. Problems arise from

- increase sputum and mucus production,

- impaired ciliary clearance of secretions in the lung,

- increases in airway reactivity,

- reduced oxygen delivery to the tissues from increased carboxyhaemoglobin levels,

- harmful effects of nicotine on heart including tachycardia and vasoconstriction.

The increased risk from smoking declines after 8 weeks abstinence.[5]

Interestingly, smokers who have abstained for < 8 weeks are at increased risk of postoperative respiratory complications.

General health

- Both the Goldman Cardiac Risk Index and American Society of Anaesthesiologists (ASA) status (as indicators of poor general health) are predictive for pulmonary as well as cardiac complications.[6,7] These are discussed in Chapter 1.

Table 2.1 – Factors causing a relative increase in risk of pulmonary complications in unselected surgery.

Risk factor	Unadjusted relative risk associated with factor
Smoking	3.4
Poor general health ASA > II	1.7
Age > 70	1.9–2.4
Obesity	1.3
COPD	2.7–3.6

Adapted from Ref. 9.

- Indeed, postoperative respiratory compromise often accompanies cardiac dysfunction and vice versa, and is a reflection of the complex relationship between cardiac and respiratory pathophysiology.

Exercise capacity

- Poor exercise tolerance is strongly predictive for respiratory complications.[7,8]

Age

- Age has not been identified as independent variable predictive of increased pulmonary risk.

- Respiratory complications are more related to coexisting conditions (more common in the elderly) than directly to age.

The changes in the respiratory system and their anaesthetic implications are discussed in detail in Chapter 7.

Obesity

- Morbid obesity may predispose to ventilatory problems in the immediate postoperative period.

- However, contrary to popular belief, obesity has not been proven to be a significant risk factor predisposing to significant respiratory complications as defined above.[9,10]

- In a recent review, it was shown that obesity posed only a relative increased risk of 1.3-fold for respiratory complications (table 2.1).

One should note, however, that morbid obesity is a significant general risk factor in the surgical patient. The main problems in the morbidly obese are

- increased incidence of hypertension and ischaemic heart disease;

- mechanical respiratory problems i.e. decreased compliance and functional residual capacity, especially when supine;

- increased incidence of perioperative infection including wound and respiratory infections;

- increased incidence of abdominal wound dehiscense;

- increased rate of DVT;

- increased oesophageal reflux leading to increased risk of perioperative gastric aspiration.

Chronic obstructive pulmonary disease

- Patients with chronic obstructive pulmonary disease (COPD) are at increased risk of postoperative respiratory complications, the level of increased risk related to the severity of the lung disease.[9] Hypercapnia is particulary ominous.

- Patients with COPD should be optimised prior to surgery with the usual therapies and those with acute exacerbations should be deferred until treated.

Asthma

- Studies conflict over whether asthma increases the risk of respiratory complications as defined above.

- The emergency patient presenting with severe, symptomatic bronchospasm, however, is a serious challenge necessitating aggressive treatment with bronchodilators. Airway instrumentation in these patients may precipitate intractable bronchospasm.

SURGERY-RELATED FACTORS

Anatomical site of surgery

Even with the patient-related factors described above taken into account, the anatomical site of surgery remains *the most important predictor of respiratory risk:*[9]

- The risk of pulmonary complications is directly related to the proximity of the incision to the diaphragm (table 2.2).

Table 2.2 – Effect of surgical site on postoperative pulmonary complications.

Anatomic site of surgery	Mean incidence of pulmonary complications (%)
Thoracic	23
Upper abdominal	22
Lower abdominal	9
Other	5
Laparoscopic	0.3–0.4

Adapted from Ref. 9.

- Respiratory complications are rare if surgery is outside the thorax or abdomen.[9]

Duration of surgery

- Surgery longer than 3 h duration increases the likelihood of respiratory complications by 1.6–5.2-fold.[11,12]

- Thus, in those patients with significant predictors of respiratory risk, one should aim for as short a procedure as possible, ideally performed by the most efficient surgeon.

General anaesthesia and muscle relaxants

- The use of general as opposed to epidural or spinal anaesthesia multiplies the respiratory risk by 1.2 to 3 times (table 2.3).[9]

- The use of muscle relaxant pancuronium in one study resulted in more than a 3-fold increase in respiratory complications when compared to the use of atracurium or vecuronium.[13] Complications probably arose through inadequate reversal, causing hypoventilation and a reduced ability to cough. The authors, therefore, recommended that pancuronium should be avoided in high–risk respiratory patients.

Preoperative assessment

This includes history, clinical examination, and relevant investigations:

- Patients should be asked about dyspnoea, productive or chronic cough, and exercise tolerance.

- Physical findings on examination, predictive of complications, include all those signs of acute and chronic lung disease including reduced air entry, percussive dullness, and wheezes or crackles.

Table 2.3 – Other surgical factors affecting pulmonary risk.

Risk factor	Site of surgery	Unadjusted relative risk associated with factor
Surgery > 3 h duration	Unselected	1.6–5.2
	Thoracic or abdominal	3.6
General anaesthesia	Unselected	1.2–~
	Thoracic or abdominal or vascular	2.2–3.0
Use of muscle relaxants	Unselected	3.2

Adapted from Ref. 9.

PULMONARY FUNCTION TESTING

The role of pulmonary function testing (PFT) is controversial. It is generally agreed that PFTs

- can detect the presence or absence of pulmonary disease;

- can determine the types of defect present; i.e. restrictive, obstructive, or diffusion defect;

- can grade the extent or severity of the defect;

- are highly reproducible;[14]

- correlate with all cause mortality.[14]

Historically, early studies on PFT were based on patients undergoing thoracic surgery for diseases including lung cancer and tuberculosis, and cut-off thresholds were established below which surgery was deemed contraindicated. Over time these values have subsequently been applied to non-thoracic surgical populations.

It is now gaining acceptance that low values only indicate the severity of current disease, but do not reliably predict complications or outcome.[9]

For example, one study[15] attempted to determine if severe airflow obstruction reliably predicted the incidence of postoperative complications, by comparing patients undergoing abdominal surgery who had significant airflow obstruction with forced expiratory volume 1 (FEV1) < 40% with a group of controls. They found that airflow obstruction only predicted postoperative bronchospasm. Outcome parameters were not different between the two groups:

- The important question is whether PFT adds to the information already gained from clinical assessment. Many authors do not believe they do, as preoperative history and respiratory examination is more sensitive and specific than abnormal preoperative spirometry.[8]

- In addition, in studies that have compared both clinical assessment and PFTs, clinical findings are more predictive of respiratory complications than are PFTs.[8,16,17]

- A review on this subject in 1989[18] concluded that there were numerous methodological limitations in existing studies that prevented them from concluding that PFTs helped to predict those at risk of pulmonary complications.

- More recently, PFTs have been shown to have inconsistent and variable predictive value.[9]

There is no evidence that PFTs improve the ability to identify patients at risk who have no clinical findings suggestive of pulmonary disease on history or examination.

However, it must be emphasised that although not definitely predictive of respiratory complications, PFTs do provide an indication of disease severity and this may prompt further optimisation and direction into risk reduction strategies, which may contribute to an improved outcome.

PFTs to determine suitability for surgery

Some advocate PFTs as a tool to identify those patients at such high risk that surgery should be avoided (see table 2.4 for commonly quoted thresholds).

This philosophy is increasingly being refuted for the following reasons:

- The accuracy and meaning of predicted postoperative spirometry values have been called into question (see above).

- Patients with PFTs suggestive of extreme risk are increasingly being shown to have an acceptable rate of pulmonary complications. This is because recent developments in risk reduction strategies have improved outcomes.

- Lung volume reduction surgery as a treatment for end stage emphysema in patients with spirometry values that hitherto were below previously defined cut-off thresholds is increasingly accepted (see below).

- One study[2] studied 107 patients undergoing surgery with an FEV1 < 50% and FEV1/forced vital capacity (FVC) ratio of <70%; postoperative respiratory complications occurred in only 29% of the patients, and there was only one death amongst 97 which underwent non-cardiac procedures.

There is still, however, a general consensus that all patients undergoing lung resection surgery should have PFTs performed. The reasons often cited include:

- To provide a baseline with which to compare postoperative values.

Table 2.4 – Preoperative spirometry with previously reported thresholds for increased pulmonary risk.

True volume	Percentage of predicted volume achieved	
	FVC%	High risk if < 70%[8]
	FEV1%	High risk if < 70%[8]
	FEV1/FVC%	High risk if < 65%[25]
Predicted postoperative volume	*Percentage of predicted postoperative volume*	
ppoFEV1 High risk < 800 ml	ppoFEV1%	High risk < 40%[19]

Percentage predicted volumes achieved based on population normals for age, sex and height.
Adapted from Refs 9, 19, 26.

- To attempt to predict who will not tolerate lung resection. Predicted postoperative values are derived from an estimation of the number of functional lung units expected to remain after surgery.

- The most widely accepted threshold for lung resection surgery has been a predicted postoperative FEV1 (ppoFEV1) > 800 ml[19] (table 2.4).

- The accuracy of these predictive models have been questioned recently in studies that have compared predicted with actual postoperative values[20,21] and showed that the predictions tended to be overly pessimistic and overestimated the loss of functional lung units. In addition, as patients recovered in the months following surgery, their spirometry results progressively improved.

Lung volume reduction surgery – confounding the PFTs

In lung volume reduction surgery, bilateral wedges of hyperinflated lung are resected to improve elastic recoil pressure and diaphragm position and function. The procedure is rapidly gaining acceptance as therapy for patients with

- end stage emphysema, including even those so severe as to be listed for lung transplantation,

- severe emphysema and malignancy (which previously would have been assessed as inoperable on the basis of spirometry results).

These patients typically have FEV1 < 35% or < 0.5 l and may also be ventilator dependant. In one study, FEV1 ranged from 0.23 to 0.5 l. Here dyspnoea improved in 89% of patients and mean FEV1 improved by 51% and FVC increased by 56%.[22]

Thus, there is now increasing evidence that PFTs should not be used to deny patients' surgery, which in the case of lung malignancy may potentially be curative.[9]

How should we select which patients should undergo PFT?

The American College of Physicians recommendations published in 1990[22] and the recent review by Smetana[9] suggest that PFT be limited to the following patient groups:

- All patients undergoing lung resection surgery.

- Patients undergoing thoracic, cardiac, or upper abdominal surgery who also either have a history of smoking or symptoms of cough, dyspnoea, or unaccountable exercise intolerance.

- Patients undergoing head and neck, orthopaedic or lower abdominal surgery with unexplained dyspnoea or pulmonary symptoms.

- Patients with COPD or asthma to determine if their airflow obstruction is optimised.

ARTERIAL BLOOD GAS ANALYSIS

The American College of Physicians recommends blood gas analysis in patients with a history of dyspnoea and tobacco use who are undergoing upper abdominal or coronary artery surgery.[23]

Hypercapnia

A number of small studies have suggested that a $pCO_2 > 45$ predisposes to pulmonary complications.[24] However, all those with high pCO_2 also had substantial airflow obstruction on spirometry and could be more identified more easily by this less invasive method.

In patients undergoing lung volume reduction surgery or lung resection, hypercapnia is not predictive for postoperative pulmonary complications.

Arterial pO_2

In the study by Nunn[25] in 1988, dyspnoea at rest was more predictive than a low pO_2 for identifying those at increased risk of postoperative ventilation.

Further reading

Johnson BD, Beck KC, Zeballos RJ. Advances in pulmonary laboratory testing. *Chest* 1999; **116**: 1377–87.

Ferguson MK. Preoperative assessment of pulmonary risk. *Chest* 1999; **115 (5 suppl.)**: 58S–63S.

Doyle RL. Assessing and modifying the risk of postoperative pulmonary complications. *Chest* 1999; **115 (5 suppl.)**: 77S–81S.

References

1. Lawrence VA, Hilsenbeck SG, Mulrow CD, Dhanda R, Sapp J, Page CP. Incidence and hospital stay for cardiac and pulmonary complications after abdominal surgery. *J Gen Intern Med* 1995; **10**: 671–8.

2. Kroenke K, Lawrence VA, Theroux JF, Tuley MR. Operative risk in patients with severe obstructive pulmonary disease. *Arch Intern Med* 1992; **152**: 967–71.

3. Pedersen T, Eliasen K, Henriksen E. A prospective study of risk factors and cardiopulmonary complications associated with anaesthesia and surgery: risk indicators of cardiopulmonary morbidity. *Acta Anaesthesiol Scand* 1990; **34**: 144–55.

4. Gracey DR, Divertie MB, Didier EP. Preoperative pulmonary preparation of patients with chronic obstructive pulmonary disease: a prospective study. *Chest* 1979; **76**: 123–9.

5. Warner MA, Offord KP, Warner ME, Lennon RL, Conover MA, Jansson-Schumacher U. Role of preoperative cessation of smoking and other factors in postoperative pulmonary complications: a blinded prospective study of coronary artery bypass patients. *Mayo Clin Proc* 1989; **64**: 609–16.

6. Lawrence VA, Dhanda R, Hilsenbeck SG, Page CP. Risk of pulmonary complications after elective abdominal surgery. *Chest* 1996; **110**: 744–50.

7. Gerson MC, Hurst JM, Hertzberg VS, Baughman R, Rouan GW, Ellis K. Prediction of cardiac and pulmonary complications related to elective abdominal and non-cardiac thoracic surgery in geriatric patients. *Am J Med* 1990; **88**: 101–7.

8. Williams-Russo P, Charlson ME, MacKenzie CR, Gold JP, Shires GT. Predicting postoperative pulmonary complications: is it a real problem? *Arch Intern Med* 1992; **152**: 1209–13.

9. Smetana GW. Preoperative pulmonary evaluation. *N Engl J Med* 1999; **340**: 937–44.

10. Phillips EH, Carroll BJ, Fallas MJ, Pearlstein AR. Comparison of laparoscopic cholecystectomy in obese and non-obese patients. *Am Surg* 1994; **60**: 316–21.

11. Brooks-Brunn JA. Predictors of postoperative pulmonary complications following abdominal surgery. *Chest* 1997; **111**: 564–71.

12. Celli BR, Rodriguez KS, Snider GL. A controlled trial of intermittent positive pressure breathing, incentive spirometry, and deep breathing exercises in preventing pulmonary complications after abdominal surgery. *Am Rev Respir Dis* 1984; **130**: 12–15.

13. Berg H, Viby-Mogensen J, Roed J *et al*. Residual neuromuscular block is a risk factor for postoperative pulmonary complications: a prospective, randomised, and blinded study of postoperative pulmonary complications after atracurium, vecuronium, and pancuronium. *Acta Anaesthesiol Scand* 1997; **41**: 1095–103.

14. Kimball WR. The role of spirometry in predicting pulmonary complications after abdominal surgery progressing toward an answer. *Anesthesiology* 1999; **90**: 353–9.

15. Warner DO, Warner MA, Offord KP, Schroeder DR, Maxson P, Scanlon PD. Airway obstruction and perioperative complications in smokers undergoing abdominal surgery. *Anesthesiology* 1999; **90**: 372–9.

16. Kroenke K, Lawrence VA, Theroux JF, Tuley MR, Hilsenbeck S. Postoperative complications after thoracic and major abdominal surgery in patients with and without obstructive lung disease. *Chest* 1993; **104**: 1445–51.

17. Cain HD, Stevens PM, Adaniya R. Preoperative pulmonary function and complications after cardiovascular surgery. *Chest* 1979; **76**: 130–5.

18. Lawrence VA, Page CP, Harris GD. Preoperative spirometry before abdominal operations: a critical appraisal of its predictive value. *Arch Intern Med* 1989; **149**: 280–5.

19. Olsen G, Block A, Swenson E *et al.* Pulmonary function evaluation of the lung resection candidate: a prospective study. *Am Rev Respir Dis* 1975; **111**: 379–87.

20. Bolliger C, Perruchoud A. Functional evaluation of the lung resection candidate. *Eur Respir J* 1998; **11**: 198–212.

21. Larsen K, Svendsen U, Milman N *et al.* Cardiopulmonary function at rest and during exercise after resection for bronchial carcinoma. *Ann Thorac Surg* 1997; **64**: 960–4.

22. Eugene J, Dajee A, Kayaleh R *et al.* Reduction pneumoplasty for patients with a forced expiratory volume in 1 second of 500 millilitres or less. *Ann Thorac Surg* 1997; **96**: 894–900.

23. American College of Physicians. Preoperative pulmonary function testing. *Ann Intern Med* 1990; **112**: 793–4.

24. Milledge JS, Nunn JF. Criteria of fitness for anaesthesia in patients with chronic obstructive lung disease. *Br Med J* 1975; **3**: 670–3.

25. Nunn JF, Milledge JS, Chen D, Dore C. Respiratory criteria of fitness for surgery and anaesthesia. *Anaesthesia* 1988; **43**: 543–51.

26. Gass G, Olsen G. Preoperative pulmonary function testing to predict postoperative morbidity and mortality. *Chest* 1986; **89**: 127–35.

3

LESSONS FROM THE NATIONAL CONFIDENTIAL ENQUIRY INTO PERIOPERATIVE DEATHS

The National Confidential Enquiry into Perioperative Deaths (NCEPOD) has produced its 10th report.[1] They take the opportunity to reflect on their own contribution to improving the quality of patient care since publication of their first report in June 1990.[2]

It is also a convenient time to reflect on the issues highlighted by NCEPOD and the lessons to be learnt in the management of the high risk surgical patient.

Note: The NCEPOD considers the quality of the delivery of care and not specifically causation of death.

- Data is collected from all NHS and Defence Secondary Care Agency hospitals in England, Wales and Northern Ireland, and public hospitals in Guernsey, Jersey and the Isle of Man, as well as many hospitals in the independent sector.

- NCEPOD collects basic details on all deaths in hospital within 30 days of a surgical procedure, through a system of local reporting.

- Since the introduction of clinical governance in April 1999, participation in the confidential enquiries has become a mandatory requirement for clinicians in the NHS.

- The data collection runs from 1st April to 31st March.

- Each year a sample is selected for more detailed review.

- Questionnaires were returned by 83% surgeons and 85% of anaesthetists for the 1998/99 report.[3]

- The NCEPOD clinical coordinators, together with the advisory groups for anaesthesia and surgery, review the completed questionnaires and then aggregate the data to produce a final report.

NCEPOD does not attempt to collect denominator data or calculate mortality figures. Data submitted to the Department of Health as hospital episode statistics is used to calculate NHS Performance Indicators.

The Performance Indicators for 1998/99[3] reveal:

- 32 956 deaths in hospital within 30 days of an operative procedure.

- 24 920 after emergency surgery and 8036 after non-emergency surgery.

- A total of 2.3 million procedures★ were undertaken (of which 26% were emergencies).

- Mortality rate of 1.4% after emergency surgery.

- Mortality rate of 0.5% after non-emergency surgery.

NCEPOD does tell us something about the distribution of these deaths:[1]

- the vast majority of patients are elderly; 70% of deaths occurred in patients > 70 years;

- 94% of patients have a coexisting medical disease;

- death occurs within 5 days of an operation in almost half of the patients reported.

Most of the recommendations taken from the 10 reports and presented below represent nothing more than common sense and good clinical practice. Many of the recommendations have been repeated over and over again.

NCEPOD RECOMMENDATIONS

Facilities

Individual clinicians efforts to provide the level of care they know is required for the high risk surgical patient is often frustratingly thwarted by lack of facilities. NCEPOD has helped identify these shortcomings. One of the major lessons to be learnt is that to provide the highest quality of care for these patients, acute surgical services may need to be concentrated on fewer well staffed and resourced hospitals.[4]

★ Definition of procedures used for Performance Indicators is not directly comparable to the definitions used by NCEPOD.

- A dedicated emergency theatre and recovery should be staffed and available 24 h a day. The aim should be to deal with emergency cases during the working day and avoid out of hours operating.[1,5–7]

- There should be easy access to a high dependency unit (HDU) and intensive care unit (ICU) on a single site.[2,7,8]

- An orthopaedic trauma theatre operating during the day with senior staff.[9]

- Elderly patients should not have to wait more than 24 h (once fit) for operation.[10] When a decision to operate is taken there should be a commitment by the clinicians and adequate facilities available to provide appropriate critical care post-operatively.[10]

- Local protocols should be in place to ensure immediate access to blood and blood products.[11]

- CT scanning and availability of neurosurgical consultation should be available in any hospital receiving trauma patients.[9]

- A fibreoptic laryngoscope should be available with trained and nominated staff able to use it.[12]

- Children's services should be concentrated to avoid occasional practice. Local arrangements should be in place for the skilled transport of critically ill children when appropriate.[1]

- An arbitrator/coordinator should exist to ensure emergency cases are prioritised appropriately and emergency theatre space is utilised efficiently.[7]

Personnel

It is clear that the high risk surgical patient should be directly cared for by experienced senior anaesthetists and surgical members of staff. This recommendation has been one of the cornerstones of the NCEPOD reports over the years:[7–10]

- In the most recent NCEPOD report[1] of the cases sampled 59% of anaesthetics were given by a consultant and 52% of operations were performed by a consultant surgeon.

- Consultant presence in these cases has changed little since the first report.[2]

- Comparing NCEPOD 2000[1] to NCEPOD 1990[2] fewer of the sampled patients are anaesthetised or operated on by junior trainees. However there is now a trend towards a greater reliance on non-consultant career grade (NCCG) anaesthetists and surgical members of staff.

It may on occasions be appropriate or unavoidable that consultants cannot be directly involved in patient care. At the very least the consultant has a vital role in providing advice, support and making crucial decisions:[5,9]

- NCEPOD 2000[1] reported that only 5% of cases had no consultant surgeon involvement.

- Disappointingly anaesthetists sought advice from a colleague who was not present during the anaesthetic in 15% of cases.[1]

There are a number of reasons why senior help may not be requested for the high risk patient:

- Insufficient experience to identify the at risk patient.

- Inability to recognise personal limitations.

- Lack of familiarity with local procedures.

- Practical barriers to communication.

- Poor understanding of personal limits of responsibility.

Though these are mainly personal shortcomings senior clinicians should ensure that the system within their hospital is robust enough to ensure these individual limitations do not compromise patient safety and good practice.

NCEPOD does provide some practical lessons to enable us to achieve the recommendation[8] of matching senior surgical and anaesthetic skills to the condition of the patient.

Supervision

- Ensure local guidelines are in place, so trainees are clear when to ask for help.[8,9]

- National or regional guidelines may be preferable to avoid confusion when trainees rotate between hospitals.[8]

- Guidelines are particularly important in paediatrics, to prevent occasional practice, ensure practitioners retain skills and to promptly identify children that require specialist care and transfer.[1,2]

Communication

- All staff (including consultants) must be aware of their limitations and work in an environment where they are encouraged to and are comfortable with asking for help.[5]

- Anaesthetists should be consulted as opposed to informed about cases.[1]

- Encourage a team approach between surgeons, anaesthetists and physicians for complex cases.[6]

- Ensure there is adequate communication between specialties and between grades of staff within a specialty.[11]

- 'Who to call', 'When to call' and 'How to call' for help should be easily available and clearly understood.[1,7]

Staff availability

- All staff covering emergencies should be free from other commitments and easily available.

- Emergency theatre sessions should be staffed by consultants.[1,7,8]

Locums and NCCG anaesthetists and surgeons

- Ensure NCCG doctors within the hospital are aware of their role and limit of responsibility. They should have equal access to supervision, involvement in audit and opportunities for continued professional development.[1]

- Supervising consultants should be aware of the abilities of locum doctors before appointment.[5]

- Extra effort and vigilance is required to ensure that locums are appraised of local guidelines and afforded the same degree of supervision and support as other members of staff.[5,11]

The Royal College of Anaesthetists provides guidance on the level of supervision of doctors in training.[13] It highlights the statement from the Clinical Negligence Scheme for Trusts (CNST) which increases the statutory requirement to ensure that doctors taking up post in a new hospital are adequately trained and competent to fulfil the role for which they have been employed. There is now a requirement for supervisors to list technical skills new doctors are expected to perform and, in turn, for the new doctors to indicate their competence to perform the specific tasks. A supervised training programme must rectify any deficiencies in initial, or continuing competence.

Pre-operative assessment and preparation

In the 10 years that NCEPOD has reported the profile of patients dying within 30 days of their operation has changed.[1]

Patients are more likely to be older, have undergone an urgent operation, be of poorer physical status and have a coexisting cardiovascular or neurological disorder.

Adequate pre-operative assessment and preparation for theatre is vital in the management of the high risk surgical patient.

The management of the patient at this time will greatly influence the subsequent outcome of the operation and it is crucial that appropriate care is given and appropriate decisions made to prevent avoidable morbidity and mortality.

- The decision to operate and when not to operate should be made by consultants.[2,12] It is important that there is direct communication between consultant surgeon and anaesthetist and decisions are made jointly.[1]

- NCEPOD has frequently referred to the problem of operations being performed on moribund patients or where the objective of surgery is unclear.[2,12] These patients clearly need a consultant evaluation and a sensitive but honest approach to the patient and relatives. Too often hasty decisions to opt for surgery are made without fully considering their ramifications.

- If the decision to operate or not is contra to that of the patient or relatives, having a mechanism to allow discussion with consultant colleagues from the same or allied specialty can be invaluable in reassuring the patient and relatives that an appropriate decision has been made.

- NCEPOD has highlighted the need to provide junior members of staff with guidance on when to ask for help.[7] NCEPOD has indicated the inadequacies and inconsistencies of the ASA classification if used as an assessment tool.[1] The ASA classification may not on its own be an adequate trigger for alerting inexperienced doctors to a high risk patient. NCEPOD suggested that the use of the P-POSSUM score should be more widespread.[10]

- The importance of avoiding rushing patients to theatre before adequate resuscitation is a recurring theme of NCEPOD.[2,8] Emergency patients invariably require appropriate fluid resuscitation prior to theatre. In some patients this can safely be undertaken on the ward. In other patients, particularly the elderly, this may require a critical care environment and appropriate invasive monitors.[1,7]

- Poor understanding of fluid management especially in the elderly is often cited as a contributing factor in NCEPOD cases.[6-8,10] The use of pre-operative critical care services for resuscitation and pre-operative preparation may well avoid the need for lengthy post-operative critical care.[7]

- Finding a critical care bed pre-operatively in many hospitals may be impossible. The ability to utilise theatre recovery beds prior to surgery and the development of critical care outreach services may be a short-term solution.

- Whatever the particular local solution it is important to have a mechanism in place to allow patients to be adequately resuscitated in an appropriate environment by knowledgeable staff.

- Starting a high risk case without first identifying adequate critical care facilities post-operatively is to be avoided.[6] Consultation with colleagues who control these beds at the earliest opportunity is essential. It is not always easy to identify those patients who require HDU care. CEPOD has called for simple nationally agreed criteria to help assess the need for HDU care.

- Over the 10 years of NCEPOD the percentage of patients with coexisting medical disorders has increased from 89% to 94%.[1] Cardiac disorders have increased from 54% to 66%. NCEPOD suggest that Echocardiography should be available and used more widely in pre-operative assessments.[1] For complex medical disorders the advice of a specialist physician may be invaluable. NCEPOD would like to see hospitals develop an organisational structure to allow prompt medical review should it be required.[1]

- Thromboembolic complications continue to be a major cause of morbidity and mortality. CEPOD has recognised this in all its reports and highlighted the inconsistent nature of prophylactic measures. It recommends the development of guidelines and clear definition of responsibility for implementing prophylactic measures. The guidelines need to be audited regularly to ensure compliance and efficacy.[1,7,8]

- Individuals dealing with high risk patients in the pre-operative period should be aware of the importance of thromboembolis prophylaxis.

Audit

CEPOD recognises that audit can be a useful tool locally to help improve the management of high risk surgery. There is a lack of consistency in the participation in audit both between hospitals and within surgical specialties and anaesthesia.

Of cases sampled for NCEPOD 2000[1] 1/3 of deaths were reviewed by anaesthetists and 3/4 of deaths reviewed by surgeons, this was unchanged from NCEPOD 1990.[2]

In an effort to improve local practice NCEPOD would recommend:

- Improved access to notes, especially of deceased patients.[1]
- More post-mortem examinations.[9]

- Better communication between pathologists and clinicians.[11]

- Regular morbidity and mortality review meetings. Ideally these should be multidisciplinary meetings to enhance the working relationships of surgeon, anaesthetist and physician.[1]

- Ensure all members of staff participate equally in audit.[1]

In the light of public concern over organ retention following post-mortem examination there is rightly greater rigour now required for the consent to post-mortem examination. Details of the consent process are beyond the scope of this book. The Department of Health (DOH) has published interim guidance on consent for post-mortem examinations.[14] In this guidance they also echo the recommendations from NCEPOD in emphasising the importance of post-mortem examination to improving clinical care and maintaining standards.

In the 10 years that NCEPOD has reported it is clear that the rate of change is often slow. Many of the lessons continue to be repeated and are not always heeded. Both managers and clinicians need the commitment backed up with resources to implement changes in practice. In their introduction to the current report, Ingram and Hoile state 'We believe that future change will depend on money, manpower, mentality and mentoring.'[1]

NCEPOD DEFINITIONS

Admission category

Elective – at a time agreed between the patient and the surgical service.

Urgent – within 48 h of referral/consultation.

Emergency – immediately following referral/consultation, when admission is unpredictable and at short notice because of clinical need.

Classification of operation

Emergency – immediate life-saving operation, resuscitation simultaneous with surgical treatment. Operation usually within 1 h.

Urgent – operation as soon as possible after resuscitation. Operation within 24 h.

Scheduled – an early operation but not immediately life-saving. Operation usually within 3 weeks.

Elective – operation at a time to suit both patient and surgeon.

Further information

NCEPOD website: www.ncepod.org.uk

References

1. Then and now. *The 2000 report of the National Confidential Enquiry into Perioperative Deaths.* NCEPOD, London, 2000.

2. Campling EA, Devlin HB, Lunn JN. *The report of the National Confidential Enquiry into Perioperative Deaths 1989.* NCEPOD, London, 1990.

3. Quality and performance in the NHS: NHS Performance Indicators. *NHS Executive,* July 2000.

4. Ingram GS. The lessons of the National Confidential Enquiry into Perioperative Deaths. *Ballieres Clin Anaesthesiol* 1999; **13 (3)**: 257–66.

5. Campling EA, Devlin HB, Hoile RW, Lunn JN. *The report of the National Confidential Enquiry into Perioperative Deaths 1990.* NCEPOD, London, 1992.

6. Devlin HB, Hoile RW, Lunn JN. One case per consultant surgeon or gynaecologist. *The report of the National Confidential Enquiry into Perioperative Deaths 1993/1994.* NCEPOD, London, 1996.

7. Campling EA, Devlin HB, Hoile RW, Ingram GS, Lunn JN. *Who operates when? A report by the National Confidential Enquiry into Perioperative Deaths 1995/1996.* NCEPOD, London, 1997.

8. Campling EA, Devlin HB, Hoile RW, Lunn JN. *The report of the National Confidential Enquiry into Perioperative Deaths 1991/1992.* NCEPOD, London, 1993.

9. Campling EA, Devlin HB, Hoile RW, Lunn JN. *The report of the National Confidential Enquiry into Perioperative Deaths 1992/1993.* NCEPOD, London, 1995.

10. Extremes of age. *The 1999 report of the National Confidential Enquiry into Perioperative Deaths.* NCEPOD, 1999.

11. Gallimore SC, Hoile RW, Ingram GS, Sherry KM. Deaths within 3 days of surgery. *The report of the National Confidential Enquiry into Perioperative Deaths 1994/1995.* NCEPOD, London, 1997.

12. Gray AJG, Hoile RW, Ingram GS, Sherry KM. Specific types of surgery and procedures. *The report of the National Confidential Enquiry into Perioperative Deaths 1996/1997.* NCEPOD, London, 1998.

13. *The CCST in Anaesthesia I: General Principles – A Manual for Trainees and Trainers.* July 2000. The Royal College of Anaesthetists.

14. *Organ Retention: Interim Guidance on Post-mortem Examination.* Department of Health, 2000.

4

ANALGESIA FOR THE HIGH RISK PATIENT

In years past severe pain was accepted as an inevitable consequence of trauma and surgery and little effort was made to provide adequate pain relief in the majority of unfortunate patients:

- Whilst adequate pain relief is a laudable objective from the humanitarian perspective, modern understanding of the pathophysiological effects of pain makes appropriate pain relief a primary objective in avoiding the common morbidities associated with surgery.

- The patient who is at 'high risk' either because of the trauma of their surgery or their poor physiological reserve therefore requires effective pain relief to avoid these potentially lethal complications.

- If this is not achieved, then these are the patients most likely to slide down the slippery slope to critical illness.

Modern approaches to the management of acute pain rely heavily on two analgesic techniques, patient controlled analgesia (PCA) using an opioid self-administered in small doses by the patient, and epidural analgesic techniques. At present there is no evidence supporting a reduction in morbidity using PCA. Epidural techniques however have been demonstrated to confer a number of benefits[1–3] and as such would seem to be the analgesic method of choice in the 'high risk' patient. Other local anaesthetic techniques used occasionally by acute pain teams may also be of benefit. Some aspects of local anaesthetic techniques are discussed in Chapter 5. The skills of a multidisciplinary acute pain service (APS) are essential to ensure optimal pain management is achieved in 'high risk' patients.

THE ROLE OF THE ACUTE PAIN SERVICE

APSs developed in response to the joint colleges' report 'Pain after Surgery' (Royal College of Surgeons and College of Anaesthetists 1990) which highlighted the poor record and lack of progress in postoperative pain management over the previous 50 years.[4] In order to improve pain management and safely introduce new techniques onto general wards, such as PCA and epidural infusions, the report recommended setting up APS led by a named consultant and a specialist nurse practitioner. Services differ slightly in structure depending upon the needs of the particular hospital but all work to the same priorities in ensuring the attainment of certain levels of good practice by the implementation of guidelines and protocols supported by education programmes and by the provision of clinical support to advise and direct patient management at ward level. In 'high risk' patients it may be worthwhile, when possible, to discuss pain management with members of the service in advance of the event.

THE PATHOPHYSIOLOGY OF ACUTE PAIN

Acute pain results from injury or inflammation and generally has a biologically useful function. This function is protective by allowing healing and repair to occur.[5] The pathophysiological effects of acute pain are summarised in figure 4.1. Many patients experience acute pain as a result of surgery.

- The effect of an anaesthetic is to lower the functional residual capacity (FRC; the volume of gas remaining in the lung at the end of normal expiration) of the lung.

- In elderly patients or those with concurrent lung disease the FRC may fall below the closing volume (the volume of gas in the lung below which small airways begin to close) of the lung leading to areas of atelectasis.[6]

- This situation may be made worse by sputum retention as a result of prolonged surgery and in such circumstances atelectasis may develop in younger patients.

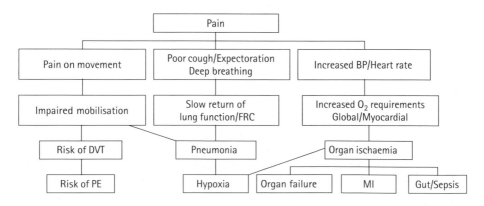

Figure 4.1 – The pathophysiology of acute pain.

- An adequate cough and ability to deep breathe is essential during the early postoperative period if these effects are to be reversed.

- This cannot generally be achieved following major abdominal or thoracic surgery without adequate analgesia and indeed the situation may worsen further if cough is inadequate as this will lead to further sputum retention, airway closure and ultimately pneumonia.

- Hypoxaemia as a result of this process will jeopardise the function of other organs. Increased myocardial oxygen requirements due to the increase in heart rate and/or blood pressure seen in the patient in pain may not be met if the patient is hypoxic.

- This may precipitate myocardial ischaemia or lead to a perioperative myocardial infarction.

- Hepatic and renal function may be compromised and ischaemia of the gut may contribute to postoperative ileus and breakdown of the gut bacterial barriers that could lead to sepsis.

- Early mobilisation can be facilitated by good pain relief and this in turn reduces the likelihood of deep venous thrombosis and pulmonary embolus and will reduce the likelihood of hypostatic pneumonia.

To promise perfect analgesia is inappropriate as this may be unachievable even with an epidural technique, thus the aims of pain management are to achieve a level of pain with which the individual can cope without distress and which will not hinder coughing and mobility. In addition pain relief should encourage and facilitate rest and normal sleep patterns whilst enabling early mobilisation and the ability of the patient to communicate with their carers. Ideally analgesic regimes should take into account periods where pain intensity is increased due to therapeutic interventions (incident pain), e.g. physiotherapy, dressing changes, etc. This is particularly important in patients with coronary artery disease who may develop myocardial ischaemia as a result.

RISK FACTORS IN PAIN MANAGEMENT

Site of injury

Pain that interferes with deep breathing and coughing confers the greatest risk to the patient and therefore the anatomical site of the surgery or injury is important when assessing risk. Thoracic surgery or injuries interfere most with the mechanics of breathing and coughing, the next most serious are upper abdominal injuries followed by lower abdominal problems and then by pain in the peripheries. When planning postoperative pain relief the site of surgery must be considered in conjunction with the patient's other risk factors.

Co-existing medical conditions

Certain medical conditions have implications for the choice of pain management. Opioid drugs are used in many analgesic techniques and can lead to respiratory depression. Patients with co-existing respiratory disease, morbid obesity, sleep apnoea and the elderly are the most at risk of respiratory depression from opioids. Although opioids are commonly used via the epidural route these patient groups may benefit greatly from the excellent analgesia that an epidural provides, particularly if the site of injury interferes greatly with respiratory function. The use of non-steroidal anti-inflammatory drugs (NSAIDs) should be avoided in patients with a number of conditions including renal failure, peptic ulceration, asthma and congestive cardiac failure and should be used with care in postoperative patients who are likely to be dehydrated. Coagulation abnormalities will preclude the use of epidural techniques and, if time and circumstances permit, consideration should be given to reversing anticoagulation to allow the use of epidural techniques in patients considered to be at high risk of problems associated with poor analgesia. Care should be taken in patients with ischaemic heart disease, whilst good analgesia protects against myocardial ischaemia the hypotension due to epidural techniques may be undesirable in the presence of a critical coronary stenosis.

THE BENEFITS OF EPIDURAL ANALGESIA IN THE HIGH RISK PATIENT

The role of good analgesia in the avoidance of morbidity is most clearly demonstrated in patients receiving epidural analgesia. Level 1 evidence (obtained from systematic review of relevant randomised controlled trials) obtained by the Australian Working party group (NHMRC) demonstrates that postoperative epidural analgesia can significantly reduce the incidence of pulmonary morbidity.[3] A review by Buggy and Smith concluded that current evidence demonstrates that epidural analgesia may facilitate early recovery and improved outcome by reducing the incidence of thromboembolic, pulmonary and gastrointestinal complications after major surgery.[1] The potential benefits of epidural analgesia in the high risk patient seem clear but the small risk of neurological complications and the potential risk of hypotension in the individual patient must be borne in mind. There is no evidence that these benefits are manifest in patients receiving parenteral opioid analgesia.

FUNDAMENTAL PRINCIPLES OF PAIN MANAGEMENT

Pain assessment

The 1990 Report of the Working Party of the Royal College of Surgeons and College of Anaesthetists recommended the systematic assessment and recording of pain during the postoperative period.[4] There is no objective measure of pain, the report of the patient is the only yardstick. If pain is not assessed expertly and regularly then the analgesic regime may be inadequate. Remember that many patients tend not to complain and will tolerate quite severe pain stoically. It is important therefore that the patient is involved in the process of assessment. The simplest tools are single-dimensional matching pain to a visual or verbal 0–10 scale with 0 – 'No Pain' and 10 – 'The Worst Pain Imaginable'.

The key points are that:

- the tool is quick and easy to use,

- the assessment is made by the patient both at rest and on movement,

- the assessment is made regularly and repeated soon after any intervention,

- the result is acted upon if the pain score is above half way up the scale.

From a therapeutic perspective patients should be comfortably able to take a deep breath and cough and as such measurement of pain on movement, deep breathing or coughing is a more important determinant of outcome than measurement of pain scores at rest. Individual assessments are crucial in *all* patients in pain to prevent the tendency towards 'blanket' prescribing.

Changes in the type or intensity of the pain being experienced by the patient should be given serious consideration as this may indicate failure of the analgesic technique, e.g. an epidural catheter falling out or becoming disconnected, or may indicate a deterioration in the patients condition. Early identification and treatment of neuropathic pain should be given consideration particularly if nerve injury is likely. Neuropathic pain is often described as 'burning' or 'shooting' and may be elicited by minimal stimulation of the affected area. It is poorly responsive to morphine which is commonly given in larger and larger doses if the diagnosis is missed. Therapy with carbamezepine or amitripyline is more appropriate and should be considered.

Multi-modal analgesia

This is also referred to as 'Balanced Analgesia' and implies the use of two or more analgesic agents in combination to effect pain relief at different places along the pain pathway. Possible analgesic agents that can be used in this way are

- opioids (higher centres and spinal cord effects via opioid receptors),

- NSAIDs (peripheral nociceptors via inhibition of cyclo-oxygenase),

- paracetamol (NSAID like effects but none of the usual side effects),

- local anaesthetics (block sodium channels and hence conduction in nerve fibres),

- tramadol and clonidine (increase activity of spinal descending inhibitory pathways by decreasing re-uptake of nor-adrenaline and 5-HT in neural synapses).

Drug combinations should be tailored to the individual depending upon circumstances and contraindications. The benefits of multi-modal analgesia are well described, better analgesia can often be achieved with greater safety and fewer side effects particularly when adjuvant analgesics are used alongside opioids when a demonstrable opioid sparing effect can be seen.

INITIAL ANALGESIA IN THE HIGH RISK PATIENT

Many patients in the 'high risk' category will present as emergency admissions either as a result of trauma or their disease process e.g. acute abdomen. Effecting good analgesia quickly should be a priority in these as in all patients. Good analgesia in the early stages helps reduce the physiological and psychological stresses brought about by trauma or disease and is particularly important in patients with ischaemic heart disease. There is no justification for withholding analgesia to facilitate clinical diagnosis, not even in the patients with acute abdominal pain. Oral analgesics are of little use as nausea or vomiting may be a feature and absorption of the drug unpredictable. Intramuscular (IM) or better still intravenous (IV) opioids are the method of choice supplemented by parenteral, rectal or 'melt' NSAIDs, unless contraindicated, or rectal paracetamol. In patients who are at higher risk of respiratory depression due to current or concurrent illness, the IV administration of an opioid to achieve analgesia is favoured as it allows careful titration of the dose against the patients response. In most patients morphine in increments of 1–2 mg or diamorphine in 1 mg increments would be the drugs of choice. It is often necessary to exceed the recommended doses for these drugs as defined in the British National Formulary, particularly if the patient has had recent exposure to other opioid drugs.

Other techniques that may be of value in this initial phase of treatment depending upon circumstances include inhalational analgesia using Entonox which is particularly useful as an adjuvant if painful interventions or movement of the patient is necessary. In some instances a simple local anaesthetic block may be of value and can easily be performed, e.g. femoral nerve block for a femoral fracture.

Early analgesia buys time until a more considered plan can be made to control the patient's pain.

ANALGESIC TECHNIQUES IN THE HIGH RISK PATIENT

APSs across the country employ a number of standard techniques to effect pain control. These techniques include PCA, epidural infusion analgesia (EIA), patient controlled epidural analgesia (PCEA), algorithm controlled opioids and a number of other local anaesthetic blocks which may be prolonged by continuous infusion via a strategically placed catheter. To ensure patient safety these techniques need a supporting package of protocols, education and clinical supervision that only a pain service can provide. If this support is not in place the general ward is not the place for a one-off epidural. For the purpose of understanding we will give here a brief description of the important techniques listed above which are well described elsewhere.

Algorithm controlled opioids

This was first described by Gould.[7] The algorithm allows the oral, IM or subcutaneous administration of morphine, usually in 10 mg doses, as regularly as every hour in response to patient need. The algorithm allows nurses greater flexibility to administer morphine in response to pain score, if respiratory rate, level of consciousness and other basic physiological parameters are acceptable. In practice a number of doses may be needed initially to achieve analgesia after which dose frequency reduces to a more 'normal' 3–4 hourly pattern.

Patient controlled analgesia

The principle here is that the patient self-titrates an opioid, most commonly morphine, in small doses, generally 1–2 mg at a time using a patient request button. Each time a dose is administered the system 'locks out' usually for 5 min during which time the request button is ineffective. Subsequent requests, after each 5 min lockout will result in further doses. This method is excellent for maintaining analgesia once achieved. Pre-loading of the patient via the IV or IM routes is mandatory to the success of the technique as using the button alone can take hours to achieve analgesia from a standing start. The patient must have the mental and physical capabilities to understand the technique and to use the button.

Epidural infusion analgesia

Placement of a catheter into the epidural space to effect analgesia has long been practised in obstetric anaesthesia. The technique is now being applied in an acute pain setting. The quality of analgesia achieved is far superior to that achieved by PCA or algorithm controlled opioids. Infusion regimes vary but usually incorporate mixtures of bupivacaine at a concentration of 0.0625–0.15% with a lipid soluble opioid (not morphine) such as diamorphine (maximum $40\,\mu$g/ml) or fentanyl (maximum $5\,\mu$g/ml). Epidural opioids are more effective when used in conjunction with a local anaesthetic to produce a synergistic analgesic action and reduce the required dose and side-effects associated with either the local anaesthetic or opioid alone. These mixtures are run at rates of up to 10 ml/h depending upon the site of insertion. Insertion of the epidural at an appropriate segmental level is important as spread of drugs within the epidural space is limited. In practice hypotension due to autonomic blockade by the local anaesthetic is a far bigger problem than respiratory depression although lowering the dose of the opioid may be wise if respiratory depression is a significant patient risk factor.

Patient controlled epidural analgesia

This is a modification of EIA. The same opioid/local anaesthetic mixtures tend to be used at similar infusion rates. The main difference is that the patient is able to self-bolus extra doses of the mixture to supplement analgesia if required. In our practice we allow a patient controlled bolus of 2 ml with a 20 min lockout to supplement background infusions of 0.125% bupivacaine with $40 \mu g/ml$ of diamorphine at up to 8 ml/h. PCEA allows greater flexibility of dose and better patient response to increases in pain intensity such as during physiotherapy.

OPTIMISING ANALGESIA IN THE HIGH RISK PATIENT

Choice of analgesic technique will depend upon the site of the surgery and other patient risk factors. The challenge is to tailor effective analgesia to each patient's requirements applying multi-modal principles using the available techniques alongside adjuvant analgesics. The objective is analgesia that is effective enough to avoid further deterioration in the patient's condition as a direct result of pain whilst avoiding side effects and complications attributable to the analgesic technique. In general the technique chosen should be used, if effective, until the patient's pain is able to be controlled on an oral analgesic combination. It is wise to ensure that this control is possible before permanently discontinuing a technique, e.g. removing an epidural catheter.

Debate still continues regarding the use of epidurals on the general postoperative ward. In our view the full benefit of epidural analgesia is only attainable if the technique is maintained until the point where oral pain control is achievable. Whilst an initial period in a high dependency unit (HDU) or intensive care unit (ICU) environment is desirable in the high risk patient whilst the patient is re-warmed and fluid management is optimised, it is inappropriate to discontinue a working epidural after only 24–36 h so that the patient can go back to the general ward. As few hospitals in the UK have HDU facilities that can cope with keeping patients for 3–4 days it is necessary to set up general wards to safely manage epidurals in order to optimise the proven clinical benefits.

ANALGESIC STRATEGIES IN THE HIGH RISK PATIENT

As site of injury is a crucial factor in pain associated risk it seems sensible to discuss basic analgesic strategies using this factor as a determinate of technique.

Pain in the peripheries

Pain in the limbs has little direct effect on breathing and coughing ability, it does however significantly limit movement. Analgesic objectives should be to promote early mobilisation to at least a sitting in chair position to minimise the chance of hypostatic pneumonia. Standard opioid techniques such as PCA or algorithm controlled opioids in combination with paracetamol and/or an NSAID would be the method of choice. A recent paper suggests that for limb injury ketorolac is as effective as morphine, produces less side effects and greater patient satisfaction.[8] The use of epidural analgesia in these patients may preclude early mobilisation due to motor blockade and postural hypotension. Other peripheral nerve blocks may be of value in producing analgesia in the early postoperative period. Some blocks, e.g. brachial plexus have a prolonged action often extending into the first or even second postoperative day and are well worth considering particularly in patients where avoidance of opioids is desirable.

Lower abdominal pain

This is most commonly a result of surgery. The majority of patients having surgery of the lower abdomen or pelvis are having elective procedures, e.g. gynaecological surgery and will cope very well with PCA or on the IM algorithm. Consideration should be given to the benefits of epidural analgesia in these patients if other risk factors exist. Morbid obesity and/or proven sleep apnoea are a clear indication for epidural analgesia as the use of opioids in these patients is fraught with risk. Supplementation of either technique with paracetamol and/or an NSAID is desirable and if an opioid technique is planned then on-table bilateral inguinal blocks give excellent adjunct analgesia in the initial postoperative period.[9]

Upper abdominal pain

Surgical incisions on the upper abdomen may well extend into the lower abdomen as a full blown laparotomy incision. Upper abdominal incisions interfere with the mechanics of breathing far more than lower abdominal incisions. A significant proportion of patients in this category will present as emergency cases with the possibility of concomitant sepsis, dehydration, electrolyte imbalance and other physiological deficits. There is clear evidence that epidural analgesia, EIA or PCEA confers a benefit in this patient group. It is the technique of choice in the majority of 'high risk' patients but there are always situations where epidural analgesia is impossible or should be used with care. These will include:

- Patient refusal (absolute contraindication).

- Infection at the site of insertion (absolute contraindication).

- Anticoagulation (consider reversal if for elective surgery).

- Fixed cardiac output states, e.g. aortic stenosis, hypertrophic obstructive cardiomyopathy, epidural blockade may precipitate profound cardiovascular collapse in these patients (use with care including full haemodynamic monitoring and postoperative intensive care).

- Systemic sepsis, epidural blockade may contribute to cardiovascular instability, there is also a theoretical increased risk of epidural abscess formation (need to balance risks carefully, consider siting epidural in early postoperative period when cardiovascular instability is less profound).

Epidural analgesia can be combined with NSAID and/or paracetamol to provide improved analgesia using multi-modal analgesia principles. Sedative drugs and parenteral opioids should be avoided if the epidural infusion contains an opioid as this increases the risk of respiratory depression.

If an epidural is out of the question other local anaesthetic blocks might warrant consideration. Intrapleural or paravertebral infusions are of use for unilateral incisions such as open cholecystectomy. A left intrapleural block has been advocated for the treatment of pancreatitis pain.[10] An infusion of local anaesthetic directly into the wound via a catheter sited during wound closure can contribute significantly to postoperative analgesia and is of value alongside standard PCA or the IM algorithm.

Thoracic pain

Pain in the thorax interferes significantly with the mechanics of breathing and coughing. Common causes are surgery and chest trauma. A well wired sternotomy wound gives surprisingly little pain but the pain following thoracotomy is very severe. Epidural analgesia is strongly recommended for most patients having thoracic surgery. The only grey area is in younger patients with non-malignant disease where an epidural, although giving excellent analgesia, is unlikely to influence a successful outcome and where neurological damage would be a major disaster. In 'high risk' patients epidural analgesia should be given a very high priority given the exclusions previously discussed. Alternative techniques which can be used alongside PCA or algorithm controlled opioids are paravertebral infusions or epiplueral infusions in which a catheter is sited outside the pleura in the paravertebral gutter under direct vision by the surgeon.[11] Thoracic epidural analgesia has clear benefits in the management of chest trauma and may reduce the need for ICU admission.

Pain in more than one location

This is a common problem following major trauma and although an epidural may be indicated to treat pain from chest trauma or a laparotomy it will not give effective analgesia for concomitant limb fractures. One strategy is to use local anaesthetic only in the epidural infusion and allow the patient to use a standard PCA to treat the pain not managed by the epidural. This strategy can also be used when epidural analgesia is inadequate due to a missed segment or when low epidural placement misses the top end of a surgical wound.

PROBLEMS ENCOUNTERED WITH EPIDURAL ANALGESIA

The complications of epidural catheter insertion are well described[6] and include epidural haematoma and abscess, IV injection of local anaesthetic and inadvertent dural tap. The risk of neurological complications either of a minor or major nature has yet to be clearly defined but must be considered when balancing the risks against the benefits of thoracic epidurals.

Itching, nausea and vomiting are all recognised side effects of epidural opioids. Though respiratory depression is rare monitoring of sedation level is mandatory. Hypotension (systolic blood pressure less than 80 mmHg) occurs in over 25% of our patients. Optimising fluid management is a major challenge and in the 'high risk' patient this may well best be achieved initially in an intensive or high dependency care environment.

Care should be taken with the timing of prophylactic heparin injections in rela- tion to insertion and removal of epidural catheters to reduce the likelihood of epidural haematoma.

Epidural analgesia is associated with the development of pressure sores particularly on the heels. This can happen even in young healthy people and nursing vigilance is essential. Debilitated patients are at higher risk of developing this complication. Strong local anaesthetic solutions administered via the epidural in theatre may be a factor in the development of these sores. A sensible precaution is to switch off epidural infusions if patients' legs are still paralysed beyond 2 h post surgery. It can be recommenced when the block has regressed enough to allow leg movement. This precaution also facilitates early detection of epidural haematoma.

INCIDENT PAIN IN THE HIGH RISK PATIENT

The acute pain experience is one that begins severely, immediately following injury, then decreases over the subsequent few days to a level that can be controlled by simple analgesics and then, in time resolving. This is not however the whole story as overlying this general downward trend are periods when pain intensity is increased by therapeutic interventions such as physiotherapy, trips to the X-ray department, dressing changes or the patients attempts to mobilise. The analgesic technique in use may need supplementation in order to cover these episodes. This is most easily achieved in the following ways:

- The use of patient controlled analgesic techniques such as PCA or PCEA. Most painful interventions can be anticipated. This allows the patient to dose himself/herself with extra morphine or epidural top ups in preparation. In this regard PCEA has distinct advantages over EIA.

- Entonox, this is a mixture of 50% oxygen in 50% nitrous oxide administered through a mask or mouthpiece via a patient activated demand valve. In essence it is patient controlled inhalational analgesia giving short duration analgesia acting for as long as the patient continues to breathe the entonox. As with IV PCA the system has a built in safety mechanism to prevent overdose if used correctly. It is essential that only the patient holds the mouthpiece so that if the patient becomes too drowsy the mask will fall away from the face. Additionally with Entonox, there is the psychological value of distraction with the act of using the device.

Further reading

Rawal N. 10 years of acute pain services – achievements and challenges. *Reg Anesth Pain Med* 1999; **24**: 68–73.

McQuay H, Moore A, Justins D. Treating acute pain in hospital. *Br Med J* 1997; **314**: 1531–5.

Carpenter RL, Abram SE, Bromage PR *et al.* Consensus statement on acute pain management. *Reg Anesth* 1996; **21**: 152–6.

References

1. Buggy D, Smith G. Epidural anaesthesia and analgesia: better outcome after major surgery? *Br Med J* 1999; **319**: 530–1.

2. Rodgers A, Walker N, Schug S *et al.* Reduction of postoperative mortality and morbidity with epidural or spinal anaesthesia: results from overview of randomised trials. *Br Med J* 2000; **321**: 1493–7.

3. National Health and Medical Research Council Report. *Acute Pain Management: The Scientific Evidence*, NHMRC, Canberra, 1999.

4. Pain after surgery. *Report of a Working Party of the Commission on the Provision of Surgical Services.* The Royal College of Surgeons of England and the College of Anaesthetists. London, 1990.

5. Woolf CJ. Somatic pain – pathogenesis and prevention. *Br J Anaesth* 1995; **75 (2)**: 169–76.

6. Atkinson R, Rushman G, Davies N. *Lee's Synopsis of Anaesthesia*, 11th edn, 1993. London: Butterworth Heinemann.

7. Gould TH, Crosby DL, Harmer M *et al.* Policy for controlling pain after surgery: effect of sequential changes in management. *Br Med J* 1992; **305**: 1187–93.

8. Rainer HT, Jacobs P, Ng YC *et al.* Cost effectiveness analysis of keterolac and morphine for treating pain after limb injury: double blind randomised controlled trial. *Br Med J* 2000; **321**: 1247–51.

9. Bunting P, McConachie I. Ilioinguinal nerve blockade for analgesia after Caesarean Section. *Br J Anaesth* 1988; **61**: 773–5.

10. Sinatra R, Hord A, Ginsberg B, Preble L. *Acute Pain: Mechanisms and Management,* 1992. London: Mosby Year Book.

11. Richardson J, Sabanathan S, Jones J *et al.* A prospective, randomized comparison of preoperative and continuous balanced epidural or paravertebral bupivacaine on post-thoracotomy pain, pulmonary function and stress responses. *Br J Anaesth* 1999; **83 (3)**: 387–92.

5

LOCAL ANAESTHETIC TECHNIQUES

Local anaesthetic techniques are widely used in high-risk surgical patients. They may be used alone or in combination with general anaesthesia to provide anaesthesia and analgesia both intraoperatively and postoperatively. A wide variety of local anaesthetic techniques are used varying from simple techniques such as wound infiltration through field and nerve blocks to major regional anaesthesia. Infusion systems may be used to provide prolonged anaesthesia or analgesia into the postoperative period.

REGIONAL AND LOCAL ANAESTHETIC TECHNIQUES

There are a large number of nerve blocks described which can be used to provide anaesthesia or analgesia for procedures or painful conditions affecting many parts of the body. These are described in detail in other texts:

- These procedures can be associated with adverse events and it is important when performing a nerve block that the anaesthetist is familiar with the anatomy both of the nerve and also of adjacent structures, the potential adverse events specific to the procedure being performed and takes all precautions to reduce these risks to the patient.

- Use of a nerve stimulator when appropriate will increase the potential for a successful block and reduce the risk of adverse effects.

Blocks have been described which can be used to provide anaesthesia or augment anaesthesia for procedures on many areas of the body. The major advantage of local and regional techniques is that they can be used to avoid general anaesthesia for surgery, or allow a reduction in the anaesthetic or analgesic dosage. This can reduce the risk of complications, particularly postoperative respiratory tract infections, nausea and vomiting, and pain. Cardiac complications such as hypotension may be reduced when using regional anaesthesia, but there is conflicting evidence on this. It is important, however, to remember that practice and experience are important factors in the success of any technique, and that a competent general anaesthetic is preferable to the serious complications of a regional technique which has gone wrong.

Adverse events from local anaesthetic techniques may be due to the technique or the agents used:

- General risks for all techniques include the risk of local infection, haematoma and trauma to the nerve which may lead to temporary or permanent symptoms. When a local or regional technique is being used as the sole anaesthetic technique it is important to consider the adverse effect of patient stress and anxiety, which can be associated with unwanted hypertension and tachycardia.

- Other risks are specific to the block which is being performed and a knowledge of these risks is important when performing any block.

Spinal and epidural anaesthesia

These techniques are very widely performed and again are associated with potential adverse events. Hypotension is a significant effect, due to blockade of sympathetic afferents. The sympathetic afferents originate in the thoracolumbar anterior nerve roots as far as L2. Block below this level is not associated with significant hypotension, increasing block height is associated with an increasing degree of hypotension. Spinal anaesthesia, which is of more rapid onset and produces profound sensory and motor block causes more hypotension than epidural anaesthesia which is more gradual in onset and which can be more controlled by slow administration. The other adverse effects of epidural and spinal anaesthesia include headache, backache, an increase risk of pressure sores, epidural haematoma, epidural abscess and risk of cord or nerve damage. Particularly, with epidural anaesthesia the block may be insufficient to be used as the sole anaesthetic or analgesic agent.

REGIONAL BLOCKADE AND TREATMENT THAT INTERFERES WITH COAGULATION

Patients who have clotting disorders have an increased risk of haemorrhage during local and regional blockade and therefore regional techniques are often contraindicated in these patients. Patients with serious haematological and liver disease, and those with severe intercurrent disease receiving thromboprophylaxis are all at increased risk of haemorrhagic complications. Many patients receiving antiplatelet treatment or anticoagulant prophylaxis now present for surgery. These treatments are particularly common in high-risk patients and the risk of haemorrhage must therefore be balanced against the potential benefits of the use of a regional technique in each individual patient.[1]

The incidence of haematoma following regional anaesthesia is extremely low. Factors involved in reducing the risk of haematoma formation include:

- uneventful needle insertion,

- the use of smaller needle size,

- avoidance of catheter insertion where possible,

- catheter removal timed to coincide with minimal anticoagulant effect.

Most research has been into the effect of these treatments in spinal and epidural anaesthesia, although there are haemorrhagic risks in other nerve blocks.

Many high-risk patients arrive for surgery on aspirin, which has an effect on platelet cyclo-oxygenase (COX) and interferes with platelet agglutination. Other non-steroidal anti-inflammatory drugs (NSAIDs) also affect platelet COX, however, their effect appears to be less prolonged than aspirin:

- The effect of aspirin can persist for 7–10 days.

- The COX 2 inhibitor NSAIDs are reported to have no effect on platelet function.

- There have been a number of case reports published where patients have developed haematoma when undergoing regional blockade while on aspirin.

- Several large studies have failed to show an increased incidence of haematoma formation in patients on aspirin coming for regional blockade compared to those not on aspirin and the incidence is therefore very low.

- Ideally a patient should omit aspirin prior to admission for surgery for 7–10 days.

The effect of heparin on epidural anaesthesia has also been extensively studied, looking at both standard and low molecular weight heparin (LMWH).[2] There have been reports of spinal haematoma in patients receiving intravenous heparin and risk factors include vessel puncture during needle siting, heparinisation within 1 h of needle, catheter siting and concomitant aspirin therapy:

- If intravenous heparin is to be commenced following a spinal or epidural, then there should be a delay of at least 1 h between the insertion of the block and commencement of heparin.

- Catheter techniques can be safely used, but the catheter should be removed at a time when heparin activity is low.

Subcutaneous heparin is also relatively safe, with few reports of spinal bleeding. Needle insertion should not be within 4 h of the last dose, and the catheter should not be removed for at least 4 h after a dose. Patients with liver disease, receiving antiplatelet therapy, or on long-term thromboprophylaxis will require monitoring of their anticoagulant effect.

LMWH has been given in a large number of patients who undergo spinal or epidural anaesthesia. These again are associated with case reports of haematoma. LMWH alter coagulation and have a 4 h half-life of effect. At 12 h after injection, there is still antithrombotic activity with 50% of maximum anti-IXa activity. These patients have altered coagulation and it is recommended that needle placement should take place at least 12 h after the last dose of LMWH with a delay of 2 h before the next dose:

- The risk of haematoma is increased by concomitant use of aspirin or dextran.

- Single dose spinal anaesthesia may be safer than epidural, as a smaller needle is used and no catheter sited.

- If a catheter is sited, this should be removed at least 12 h after a dose of LMWH, by leaving removal to 24 h after the last dose coagulation can be normalised.

- After removal of the catheter, there should be at least a 2 h delay before the next dose.

AGENTS USED IN LOCAL AND REGIONAL ANAESTHESIA

Local anaesthetic agents are the most widely used agents in local and regional techniques, but other agents may be used to cause vasoconstriction and thus prolong their effect, such as adrenaline. Many analgesic agents have been used to augment or replace the local anaesthetic, especially in spinal and epidural techniques. These agents may all have adverse effects on the patient which must be considered.

Local anaesthetic agents

There are a large number of local anaesthetics available. These are tertiary amino esters or amides, which work by acting on the nerve cell and interfering with the transfer of sodium ions across the membrane. They thus interfere with the generation of action potentials. Different nerves are affected by different concentrations of local anaesthetics and pain, temperature and touch fibres are affected at lower concentrations than motor fibres. However, it is not possible to produce a complete sensory block in a mixed nerve fibre without producing some motor blockade.

Local anaesthetic agents affect a variety of excitatory tissues and can have effects on a variety of systems, particularly the central nervous system (CNS) and the cardiovascular system. In the CNS, inhibitory neurones are more affected than excitatory, and local anaesthetics can cause tremors and restlessness and seizures in overdose. The respiratory centre can also be affected by overdose, initially causing an increase in respiration but at higher doses respiratory depression.

Cardiovascular system effects include cardiac and peripheral effects. All local anaesthetics apart from cocaine act as vasodilators via an effect on arterioles, bupivacaine having less effect than many other agents. Cocaine acts as a vasoconstrictor. Autonomic ganglia may also be affected by local anaesthetics via an anti-muscarinic effect. Local anaesthetics also act directly on the excitatory tissue of the heart causing an increase in the refractory period, prolonged conduction time and depression of myocardial excitability. This effect has been used as an advantage in the treatment of ventricular extrasystoles, tachycardia and fibrillation with lignocaine, although lignocaine can increase the defibrillation threshold.

Local anaesthetics are metabolised in the liver. Procaine and amethocaine are also metabolised by plasma cholinesterases.

Side effects are rare from local anaesthetic agents, but toxicity can be a major risk especially:

- When an overdose is given. The dose to be given should be calculated from the safe dosage for each patient. If agents are mixed, repeated doses are given or for an infusion use, this must be calculated to be within safe limits.

- Injection into a vein. It is important to aspirate prior to and during injection of local anaesthetic and if using an infiltration technique to keep the needle moving to avoid this.

- Injection into very vascular tissue or application over mucous membrane where absorption is rapid.

- Severe hepatic impairment where metabolism and excretion may be reduced.

It is important to be familiar with and prepared to manage the effects of local anaesthetic toxicity when using as part of an anaesthetic technique. Adequate monitoring and resuscitation equipment should be available when using these agents and toxic dosage should be avoided.

Vasoconstrictor agents

Local anaesthetic agents may be used in combination with a vasopressor. These are used to counteract vasodilatation, which will slow systemic absorption of the agent and reduce bleeding in the surgical field. By slowing systemic absorption of the agent, it is possible to increase the safe dose of many but not all local anaesthetic agents and also to prolong their effect.

Adrenaline is most widely used as a vasopressor agent in combination with local anaesthetics. Despite acting as a vasoconstrictor, it is systemically absorbed and can produce a significant effect causing tachycardia, hypertension and anxiety. In dental anaesthesia, this has been shown to have a significant effect in elderly patients with hypertension who demonstrate an increased risk of tachycardia and hypertension.[3] However, it has been used safely for many years in these patients and its effect on morbidity and mortality seems to be minimal. Felypressin is an alternative vasoconstrictor used in dental practice which avoids this effect.

Many other drugs have been used in combination, either alone or in combination with local anaesthetic to provide enhanced analgesia and anaesthesia. In combination with low dose local anaesthetic, they can provide intra- and postoperative analgesia with less risk of adverse effects from use of one or other alone agent. These drugs are used commonly in as adjuvants in spinal and epidural anaesthesia, but are also effective in plexus and nerve blocks.

Opioid analgesics

These are used especially in spinal and epidural techniques to enhance the analgesic effect and also to allow a reduction in the concentration and dosage of local anaesthetic. They can be given in much smaller doses than their systemic dose and are less likely to produce respiratory depression and other side effects. Opioids given spinally work locally on the opioid receptors in the dorsal horn, but also spread more centrally within the CNS. For this reason, respiratory depression can occur, especially following intrathecal opiate administration and this may be a late complication. The rate of onset of spinal opioids is related to their lipid solubility.

Epidural opioids work both at local spinal receptors but also at supraspinal levels. Epidural opioids are absorbed into the epidural venous plexus and this is probably a major contribution to their supraspinal effect. When given epidurally, the effect is related to the lipid solubility of the opioid used:

- Lipophillic agents such as fentanyl are rapidly absorbed by surrounding fatty tissues as well as crossing the dura, thus having a rapid onset but requiring higher doses than less lipid soluble agents such as morphine.

Respiratory depression is a major complication of spinal and occasionally epidural opioids, and may occur several hours following administration. It appears to be a supraspinal effect and can be reversed by naloxone. Pruritis and urinary retention are other side effects of intrathecal and epidural use of opiates.

Other agents

These are used to augment regional anaesthesia and include clonidine, an alpha agonist. Clonidine has been used spinally and epidurally and also as part of brachial plexus and lower limb nerve blocks. It is used in combination with local anaesthetic to potentiate the effect and duration of the block:

- Clonidine is associated with hypotension and drowsiness at low dose, which could preclude its use in many high-risk patients.

- It causes less urinary retention than opiates when used spinally and epidurally.[4]

- When used in nerve blocks, clonidine prolongs and augments the local anaesthesia without significant hypotension.

BENEFICIAL EFFECTS OF REGIONAL BLOCKADE ON THE STRESS RESPONSE TO SURGERY

There is an endocrine response to surgery which causes an increase in the production of pituitary hormones and stimulation of the sympathetic nervous system. This process produces a number of metabolic effects which are generally catabolic.

The stress response is considered a contributor to patient morbidity and mortality following major surgical procedures, and ways of reducing the response have therefore been widely studied. In particular, the use of regional anaesthetic techniques and especially epidural anaesthesia have been studied in relation to their modification of the stress response.[5] This has, so far, not been extrapolated to an overall increase in survival in any study. See also Chapter 12.

BENEFITS OF SPINAL AND EPIDURAL ANAESTHESIA

These have been extensively studied and shown to have a number of potential benefits for the patient:

- **Thromboembolic effect** – Regional anaesthesia has been shown to reduce the incidence of thromboembolic complications considerably. This is especially the case following surgery to the lower limbs and pelvis. The effect is partly due to lower limb vasodilatation, inhibition of the stress response and therefore reduced platelet aggregability, alteration of tissue aggregation and inhibition factor production.[6]

- **Cardiovascular effect** – There is a reduction in hypertensive and tachycardic response to surgery with regional anaesthesia. There may be a reduction in risk of myocardial infarction or cerebrovascular accident (CVA) for patients undergoing regional anaesthesia.[7]

- **Respiratory** – There is an improvement in respiratory parameters in patients receiving regional anaesthesia compared to general anaesthesia. There is also a reduction in postoperative respiratory infections. Patients with severe chronic lung disease have been shown to suffer less postoperative respiratory complications following regional anaesthesia.[8]

- **Blood loss** – The transfusion requirements of patients undergoing a regional anaesthetic technique are reduced both intra- and postoperatively when a regional technique is used.

- **Gastrointestinal function** – This is improved by regional anaesthesia with local anaesthetic and opioid following abdominal surgery. There is a lower incidence of ileus compared to patients receiving systemic opioids or epidural opioid alone. This allows a return to early enteral nutrition and the postoperative benefits of improved nutrition for the patient.

- **Infection** – There is a reduction in overall infection rates. This is particularly the case for respiratory tract infections.

- **Postoperative recovery** – There is an improvement in patient analgesia with regional techniques.

- **Mortality rate** – Some studies have shown a reduction in mortality rates for patients undergoing regional anaesthesia, with or without general anaesthesia, however, this is not universally reported and some studies have shown a possible increase in mortality rates.

The advantages listed above have been hoped to be associated with a demonstration of shortened hospital stay and postoperative complications, but these have not been proven conclusively.

LOCAL AND REGIONAL ANAESTHESIA IN PATIENTS WITH SERIOUS INTERCURRENT DISEASE

The theoretical advantages of avoiding general anaesthesia and providing a theoretical reduction in cardiovascular and respiratory risks has made local and regional anaesthesia very popular in patients with serious coexisting disease. Groups who have been extensively investigated include the following.

Patients with cardiac disease

These patients are at risk of increased perioperative morbidity and mortality, and this is especially the case in those with recent myocardial infarct or congestive cardiac failure. Patients at risk of cardiovascular complications include patients with known ischaemic heart disease, hypertensive disease and the elderly.

Local and regional techniques are often used in this group to avoid the cardiovascular effects of general anaesthesia and they have theoretical advantages, e.g. the reduction in the hypertensive and tachycardic response to surgery.

Local anaesthetic techniques for dental and eye surgery in these patients have been used very safely. The use of adrenaline as an adjunct to dental anaesthesia has been performed safely for many years without serious clinical problems in this group of patients, although there is an increased risk of arrhythmias especially in those with congestive cardiac failure or taking digoxin.[9] There is a risk of anxiety-related problems in these patients which can counteract some of the cardiac benefits of avoidance of general anaesthesia.

Local and regional anaesthesia has also increasingly replaced general anaesthesia for carotid endarterectomy. There may be an advantage related to incidence of myocardial ischaemia for local anaesthesia compared to general anaesthesia but this is, so far, not proven.[10]

Spinal and epidural anaesthetic techniques are also used widely in these patients. There is evidence that epidural anaesthesia is safer than spinal anaesthesia:

- Spinal anaesthesia is associated with more hypotension than epidural anaesthesia and this is of rapid onset.

- In patients with cardiac risk, use of spinal anaesthesia has also been associated with an increased incidence of postoperative cardiac complication and mortality in comparison to general and epidural anaesthesia.

However, the overall message is that a recent large review of regional anaesthesia supports the view that spinal and epidural techniques are associated with reduced mortality compared to general anaesthesia used alone.[11]

Patients with severe pulmonary disease

This group of patients has an increased risk of postoperative respiratory complications and local anaesthetic techniques are often used as the treatment of choice in these patients:

- General anaesthesia has been reported as a risk factor for the development of a postoperative respiratory complication when compared with local or regional techniques.

- Patients with respiratory disease presenting for orthopaedic surgery have been shown to have reduced morbidity and mortality following regional techniques.

- There is controversy still over whether use of postoperative regional analgesia can reduce pulmonary mortality following major surgery,[12] although it appears likely to have a beneficial effect.

Patients with chronic renal failure

Local and regional techniques are both used to provide anaesthesia for formation of arterio–venous fistulae in this group of patients. Brachial plexus blocks have been shown to be very safe in these patients and are used widely for fistula formation.

Using a regional anaesthetic technique should also provide these patients with beneficial effects due to avoidance of the effects of general anaesthesia on renal blood flow and the electrolyte and water retention produced by the stress response. However, it is important to maintain a normal blood pressure and cardiac output to retain this benefit.[13]

Elderly patients

These patients frequently have a number of medical conditions that increase their perioperative risk and therefore frequently receive regional or local anaesthesia. Studies have shown beneficial effects from regional anaesthesia, particularly in orthopaedic surgery.

Orthopaedic surgery

Regional anaesthetic techniques are used widely for patients undergoing orthopaedic and trauma surgery. The benefits of a reduction in thromboembolic complications, haemorrhage, and postoperative infections have led to their use in these patients who are often at high risk due to their age and intercurrent medical problems. There is an early reduction in morbidity and mortality, although this does not always extrapolate to long-term improved survival and some studies have been unable to show any relative benefit for regional anaesthetic techniques over general.[14]

Further reading

Atanassoff PG. Effects of regional anesthesia on perioperative outcome. *J Clin Anesth* 1996; **8**: 446–55.

Hall GM, Ali W. The stress response and its modification by regional anaesthesia. *Anaesthesia* 1998; **53 (suppl. 2)**: 10–12.

References

1. Knowles PR. Central nerve block and drugs affecting haemostasis – are they compatible? *Curr Anaesth Crit Care* 1996; **7**: 281–8.

2. Horlocker TT, Heit JA. Low molecular weight heparin: biochemistry, pharmacology, perioperative prophylaxis regimens and guidelines for regional anesthetic management. *Anaesth Analg* 1997; **85**: 874–85.

3. Zhongxiang-Lim, Wengi-Geng. Tooth extraction in patients with heart disease. *Br Dental J* 1991; **170**: 451–3.

4. Gentili M, Bonnet F. Spinal clonidine produces less urinary retention than spinal morphine. *Br J Anaesth* 1996; **76**: 872–3.

5. Hall GM, Ali W. The stress response and its modification by regional anaes-thesia. *Anaesthesia* 1998; **53 (suppl. 2)**: 10–12.

6. Neimi TT, Pitkanen M, Syrjala M, Rosenberg PH. Comparison of hypoten-sive epidural anaesthesia and spinal anaesthesia on blood loss and coagulation during and after total hip arthroplasty. *Acta Anaesth Scand* 2000; **44**: 457–64.

7. Rodgers A, Walker N, Schug S *et al*. Reduction of postoperative mortality and morbidity with epidural or spinal anaesthesia: results from overview of randomised trials. *Br Med J* 2000; **321**: 1493–7.

8. Pedersen T. Complications and death following anaesthesia. *Danish Med Bull* 1994; **41 (3)**: 319–31.

9. Blinder D, Shemesh J, Taicher S. Electrocardiographic changes in cardiac patients undergoing dental extraction under local anaesthesia. *J Oral Maxillofacial Surg* 1996; **54 (2)**: 162–5.

10. Ombrellaro M, Freeman MB, Stevens SL, Goldman MH. Effect of anesthetic technique on cardiac morbidity following carotid artery surgery. *Am J Surg* 1996; **171**: 387–90.

11. Racle JP, Poy JY, Haberer JP, Benkhadra A. A comparison of cardiovascular responses of normotensive and hypertensive elderly patients following bupiva-caine spinal anesthesia. *Reg Anesth* 1989; **14 (2)**: 66–71.

12. Ballantyne JC *et al*. The comparative effects of postoperative analgesic ther-apies on pulmonary outcome: cumulative meta-analyses of randomised, controlled trials. *Anesth Analg* 1998; **86 (3)**: 598–612.

13. Burchardi H, Kaczmarczyk G. The effect of anaesthesia on renal function. *Eur J Anaesthesiol* 1994; **11**: 163–8.

14. Gilbert TB *et al*. Spinal anaesthesia versus general anaesthesia for hip frac-ture repair: a longitudinal observation of 741 elderly patients during 2 year follow-up. *Am J Orthopaed* 2000; **29 (1)**: 25–35.

6

THE CRITICALLY ILL PATIENT IN THE OPERATING THEATRE

Anaesthetic management of the critically ill patient who requires operative intervention remains a significant challenge.

These patients should always be anaesthetised by senior anaesthetists.

Such patients present to the anaesthetist from three main areas within the hospital:

1. *The accident and emergency department*
   Victims of major trauma requiring immediate operative intervention fall into two categories:

   - Major haemorrhage of any source that cannot be controlled by simple resuscitative measures such as pressure dressing and splinting may transfer to the operating theatre while active fluid resuscitation is ongoing.

   - Patients with traumatic intracranial haemorrhage resulting in increased intracranial pressure (ICP) will need urgent decompression if they are to avoid medullary 'coning'. Again such casualties may require operative intervention prior to instituting full resuscitative measures.

   Patients presenting with acute general surgical pathology of a non-traumatic nature may occasionally proceed from the accident and emergency (A&E) department straight to theatre, however, it is far more likely that there will be adequate time for some degree of resuscitation and detailed investigation on the general ward or high dependency unit (HDU) prior to surgery.

2. *The hospital ward or high dependency unit*
   Patients who have already been admitted to the ward environment may deteriorate during the course of their management. This may necessitate a more precipitous trip to the operating theatre than had originally been anticipated. It is, however, likely that a degree of resuscitative intervention will already have occurred.

3. *The intensive care unit*

    This group of patients have the advantage to the anaesthetist that, provided they have spent a number of hours on the unit, they are most likely to have all resuscitative measures in place. Mechanical ventilation has usually been instituted, together with invasive lines for both monitoring and the administration of drugs and fluid.

Clearly the corollary of this situation is that this group of patients may be profoundly 'sick' receiving multi-system support on the intensive care unit (ICU); support that should ideally continue during any trip to the operating theatre.

These then are the patients who may fall into the category of critical illness. Regardless of the source of both patient and surgical pathology the issues and principles of anaesthesia surrounding any operative procedure on them remain the same. The individual patient and his or her pathology merely alter the emphasis. The remainder of this chapter will consider these principles in some detail.

PATIENT TRANSFER TO AND FROM THE OPERATING THEATRE

The safe transfer of any patient around a hospital requires organisation and planning. Even the most urgent of transfers to the operating theatre must not be undertaken, until all steps to ensure that the patient will not be harmed by the transfer have been addressed. One needs to guard against complacency because one is 'only going down the corridor'.

The principles of safe patient transfer are the same regardless of the distance involved. There are a number of texts devoted to this topic. The Association of Anaesthetists of Great Britain and Ireland and the Intensive Care Society have published guidelines for safe patient transfer (see Further reading). These include:

-   Patient's airway must be adequately secured.

-   Ventilation must be adequate, either spontaneous or mechanical. It has been shown that manual ventilation with a bag is unpredictable and unreliable compared with a portable mechanical ventilator. Ventilate with the same modes as in ICU. Modern portable ventilators can supply positive end expiratory pressure (PEEP) vary the inspiratory : expiratory (I : E) ratio and provide other modes of respiratory support.

-   Lifting of patients on and off trolleys is a cause of inadvertent extubation. It is probably safest to temporarily disconnect the ventilator for a few seconds during movement.

-   Blood pressure (BP) must be maintained with a combination of fluids and inotropic agents. Stabilise patient before transfer, if possible.

-   Patient monitoring must be appropriate to ensure safe transfer.

- Consideration should be given to pharmacological sedation and muscle relaxation as indicated by the clinical condition.

- Communication between transferring and receiving staff should ensure safe receipt of the patient.

- One must avoid last minute panic and rush. Planning should be such as to minimise delays and waiting in theatre reception areas. Check the availability of equipment in the X-ray department before the transfer commences. Check that adequate porter services are available.

- Appropriate equipment required during the transfer includes a portable ventilator, full oxygen cylinder, equipment for reintubation, drugs – for example, sedation, paralysis, cardiac resuscitation, self-inflating bag or equivalent in the event of ventilator/oxygen supply failure and battery-powered syringe pumps if required. There is no excuse for battery-powered equipment becoming exhausted, oxygen cylinders emptying or drug syringes running out.

Pitfalls and problems

- Inadequate resuscitation. Beware of occult injuries in multiple trauma patients.

- Staff and equipment problems. Inexperienced medical or nursing staff should not be used for transferring critically ill patients.

- Appropriate technical support should be available and take responsibility for the necessary equipment.

As important as ensuring the safety of the patient to be transferred is the importance of not delaying the transfer to the operating theatre by undertaking procedures that can be performed later during the operation. For example, if a patient is exsanguinating and needs a laparotomy for abdominal trauma, there is little to be gained by spending time in the A&E department inserting an arterial line. This procedure can be performed during the laparotomy when the surgeon has begun to effect haemostasis. There is no merit in delivering a corpse with an arterial line to the operating table.

PATIENT POSITIONING

When positioning the critically ill patient there are a number of points that merit emphasis:

- The critically ill patient rarely travels alone! The number of lines, tubes and bags increases with the severity of the patient's condition. Every piece of equipment inserted into the patient is there for a reason (or time should not have been wasted inserting it) and it, therefore, must be accessible during an operative procedure.

- Patients who have come to theatre as a result of trauma may well not have had a full primary and secondary survey (as the operative procedure may constitute 'C' of the primary survey). In such cases it is vital that the presence of as yet undiagnosed fractures to any part of the spine is taken into account when moving and positioning the patient. In particular the cervical spine should stay fixed with head blocks and strapping and the patient should not be moved without formal log rolling technique being used.

- Patients who have been critically ill on the intensive care and have a significant sequestration of fluid into the extra-vascular compartments will have oedematous skin that is weakened and is prone to tearing, bruising and vulnerable to pressure injury. Every effort should be made to minimise any damage done to the skin in such cases by providing adequate support and padding to the patient's exposed extremities.

PERIOPERATIVE HYPOTHERMIA

Maintenance of body temperature is important. Although there is some limited evidence that heat generation may occur following certain types of acute injury it is far more common for the traumatised patient to present to the operating theatre cold and peripherally 'shut down'. The reasons for this are as follows:

- Following acute blood loss the cardiovascular response is profound peripheral vasoconstriction resulting in maintained perfusion of vital organs, brain, heart, lungs and kidneys at the expense of other vascular beds.

- During acute traumatic injury central mechanisms of thermoregulation are disrupted. Thus shivering is diminished or absent. Whether this is secondary to reduced oxygen delivery or a response to altered hormonal activity in the thermoregulatory centre in the brain stem is unclear.

- In order to fully assess the extent of injury in the traumatised patient it is necessary to remove clothing and leave the patient exposed during repeated examination. This is compounded by the infusion of unwarmed intravenous (IV) fluid and blood worsening the relative hypothermia.

In addition to the above problems in trauma patients, all patients undergoing major surgery are at risk of becoming hypothermic (core temperature < 36°C). Reasons include:

- reduced metabolic rate associated with anaesthesia,

- vasodilation under anaesthesia,

- abolished subclinical shivering,

- exposure,

- cold fluids used for skin preparation – which are usually allowed to evaporate,

- inadequately warmed IV fluids.

Adverse effects of perioperative hypothermia

Postoperative hypothermia has become recognised in recent years as a significant, and common problem:

- Delayed awakening due to decreased clearance of anaesthetic agents.

- Most organ function is depressed by hypothermia.

- Haemodynamic instability during rewarming – increased fluids often needed as the patient vasodilates during rewarming. The hypotension thus produced can be confused with continued bleeding.

- Oxygen consumption is increased by about 140% by shivering during rewarming. If oxygen delivery to the tissues is not able to match this increase, the oxygen debt is prolonged.

- Wound infection rates may be increased by reductions in skin blood flow.

- Cell-mediated immune function may be reduced.

- Hypothermia causes coagulopathy and a decrease in platelet count. Intra- and postoperative blood loss is increased with hypothermia, for example, the typical decrease in core temperature during hip replacement increases blood loss by about 500 ml.[1] Normalisation of clotting problems will require normalisation of temperature as well as giving clotting factors.

- Adrenergic responses are increased postoperatively in hypothermic patients – responsible for increased cardiac morbidity. There is a 55% less relative risk of adverse cardiac events when normothermia is maintained.[2] Unintentional hypothermia is associated with increased incidence of myocardial ischaemia in the postoperative period.

Note:

1. The degree of hypothermia in many of the studies cited was not that severe – 35°C. Thus, development of hypothermia after prolonged surgery is highly significant and warrants serious attention to its prevention and management.

2. Laboratories perform coagulation studies at 37°C – regardless of the temperature of the patient at the time the sample was taken. Thus, these studies may underestimate the degree of impairment of coagulopathy in the hypothermic patient – what is after all a dynamic problem *in vivo* rather than *in vitro*.

Prevention of hypothermia

All practical measures should be undertaken to minimise heat loss and maintain the patient's body temperature:

- Circle system ventilation with carbon dioxide absorber and heat and moisture exchanger in the patient circuit.

- Fluid warmer for all IV fluids.

- Warmed patient mattress.

- Insulation of all areas of the patient that do not need to be exposed for either surgical or anaesthetic access. This may be achieved by wrapping or the application of an air warming system.

VENTILATION AND AIRWAY MANAGEMENT

Most critically ill patients presenting to the operating theatre will already have some form of definitive airway control in place. Under most circumstances it would be prudent to leave this airway alone for fear of losing control in a patient who may have acquired abnormalities with their airway due to tissue swelling or trauma. If the airway is not secure, one should assume a full stomach and take appropriate precautions – assume a cervical spine injury in all trauma patients. Under certain circumstances it is appropriate to use the trip to the operating theatre as an opportunity to alter airway management. For example, patients who require ventilation on the ICU for an extended period benefit from the insertion of a tracheostomy. Although it is often possible to do this via the percutaneous route in the ICU, on occasions where technical difficulties preclude this it may be possible to combine an operative event in theatre with insertion of a tracheostomy, thus limiting patient transfers.

Ventilation of the critically ill patient should always be controlled using appropriate drugs for anaesthesia and muscle relaxation. There is no place for spontaneous ventilation in this circumstance. Controlled mechanical ventilation not only allows surgical access, it may allow optimisation of gas exchange by manipulation of minute volume and oxygenation.

Where at all possible the ventilatory strategy undertaken should attempt to avoid volutrauma and barotrauma both of which may serve to worsen any degree of acute respiratory distress syndrome (ARDS) from which the patient may be suffering. Ideally the mode of ventilation in the operating theatre and, indeed, in transit to and from the ICU or A&E should be of the same standard as can be delivered in the ICU. Pressure control ventilation with the ability to alter (reverse) the I : E ratio and to apply PEEP is ideal. Lack of ongoing ventilation with PEEP and the other lung recruitment manoeuvres taken in the ICU will result in loss of recruitment of alveoli and hypoxia. This should not be a problem for most 'normal' patients ventilated in theatre as part of anaesthesia but critically ill patients under anaesthesia are different:

- Most critically ill patients presenting for anaesthesia have significant acute respiratory disease.

- Preoperative presence of increased pulmonary vascular resistance is common in critically ill patients.

- The usual presence of diseased lungs with lesser compliance results in greater increases in peak and mean airway pressures compared to 'normal' patients under anaesthesia.

Occasionally to ensure minimal deterioration in respiratory physiology it may be necessary to move a static ICU ventilator to the operating theatre and ventilate the patient on it throughout the procedure. Under this circumstance it would be necessary to adopt a total IV anaesthetic technique.

There has for some time now been a need for transport ventilators capable of delivering appropriate modes of gas delivery for critically ill patients. Recently a number of genuinely portable machines with these facilities have become available.

CHOICE OF ANAESTHETIC AGENTS

Every available technique and drug combination has been used to anaesthetise the critically ill patient. To some extent the reader must distil his or her own technique from the many approaches that they will see during their training. The way a drug is used, for example, dose, speed of injection, etc. may be more important in many patients than the absolute choice of drug. That being said, there are, however, a number of pharmacological properties and principles that should aid in this decision-making.

Induction agents

1. **Thiopentone** (sulphur analogue of pentobarbitone): Remains the most rapidly effective drug for the induction of general anaesthesia. Rapid sequence induction for the purposes of securing the airway is best performed with Thiopentone. Thiopentone is the only induction agent that reduces the brain's metabolic requirement for oxygen and is hence

neuroprotective. It produces depression of myocardial contractility together with vasodilation resulting in a fall of BP. However, it is note-worthy that in the hypovolaemic or shocked patient the sleep dose of Thiopentone is greatly reduced as compared to the healthy patient.

2. **Etomidate** (carboxylated imidazole): The main advantage is said to be cardiovascular stability when compared to Thiopentone. It inhibits 17α, 11β hydroxylase enzymes in adrenal steroid synthesis. Therefore, it is contraindicated as an infusion due to the above adrenal suppression resulting in increased mortality in patients sedated with this agent.

3. **Propofol** (di-isopropyl phenol): Rapid onset (although a little slower than Thiopentone) and obtunds pharyngeal and glottal reflexes to a greater extent than Thiopentone. Widely used for total IV anaesthesia and ICU sedation. The hypotension produced is chiefly secondary to vasodilation rather than myocardial depression.

4. **Ketamine** (phencyclidine derivative): Sympathomimetic effects main-tain BP but the increases in heart rate (HR) and stroke volume increase myocardial work. It is profoundly analgesic and is an effective analgesic agent at subanaesthetic doses. Despite sympathomimetic effects, it may cause cardiac depression, myocardial ischaemia and collapse in shocked patients in whom catecholamine stores may be exhausted.

Opioids

The key issue is the cautious use of short acting agents. The shortest available is Remifentanil.

Advantages:

- very short acting (metabolised by plasma cholinesterase),
- no accumulation in hepatorenal failure,
- very potent,
- suitable as an adjunct to sedation,
- may reduce the need for muscle relaxants.

Disadvantages:

- must be reconstituted from powder,
- profound respiratory depression,
- must be infused,
- no postoperative analgesia,

- causes decrease in BP (decrease in SVR and myocardial contractility) – worsened in hypovolaemia.

The lack of postoperative effect of Remifentanil (said to be like 'liquid nitrous oxide') and its titratability cause many anaesthetists to prefer its use for all high risk patients. Of course, additional measures must be taken for postoperative analgesia, for example, epidural anaesthesia.

Other opioids

- Fentanyl: minimal effect on the cardiovascular system in the stable, calm patient undergoing cardiac surgery. In shocked patients exhibiting high sympathetic tone, abolition of this with Fentanyl results in a fall in BP.

- Morphine should be used with great care in the critically ill patient as it has pharmacologically active metabolites and is reliant on the liver and kidneys for its elimination.

Muscle relaxants

There are four main factors governing the choice of muscle relaxant for anaesthesia:

- *Onset* – All critically ill patients are assumed to have a full stomach. Despite recent introduction of faster onset non-depolarising drugs such as Rocuronium, Suxamethonium remains the 'gold standard' for rapidly securing the airway. If cardiac instability is a major concern, Rocuronium may be a better choice.

- *Cardiovascular effects* – Rocuronium has least cardiac effects of the relaxants followed by Vecuronium. However, the vagolytic and sympathomimetic effects of Pancuronium may make it an appropriate choice in shocked patients.

- *Termination of effect and excretion* – Agents not dependent on the kidney or liver for termination of effect sound attractive in the shocked patient but from a practical point of view few critically ill patients are 'reversed' at the end of the operation and, thus, length of action of the muscle relaxants is not a big problem.

- *Duration* – In a similar manner, short or long duration is not usually an issue.

Inhalational agents

1. **Enflurane** – Greatest degree of myocardial depression for equivalent MAC.

2. **Sevoflurane** – Less increase in cerebral blood volume. Short acting.

3. **Halothane** – Rarely used nowadays. Long acting with more active metabolites retained in body than other volatile agents with potential

for liver toxicity. Sensitises the heart to endogenous and exogenous catecholamines with the potential for arrhythmias.

4. **Isoflurane** – Impressive safety profile in large numbers of patients. Hypotension chiefly by vasodilation rather than myocardial depression. Early concerns re-coronary steal are unfounded in conventional usage.

5. **Desflurane** – Specialised delivery systems required. Short acting. Some concerns re-coronary steal.

6. **Nitrous oxide** – In normal patients mild indirect sympathetic stimulation reduces any myocardial depressant actions of N_2O. Following haemorrhage this protecting effect is lost and N_2O has the same depressant effects on the heart as Halothane. With the additional concerns re-lesser inspired oxygen concentrations and the potential for expansion of air spaces, for example, pneumothoraces, it is difficult to see a major role for N_2O in critically ill patients.

Adverse effects of anaesthesia in shocked patients

In addition to the usual adverse effects of anaesthesia the critically ill and high risk surgical patient may be at additional risk from exposure to anaesthesia:

- Anaesthesia modifies the normal compensatory response to hypoxia in animals.[3] The normal compensatory increase in cerebral and coronary blood flow does not occur under volatile anaesthesia. Thus, in the critically ill patient who becomes hypoxic, anaesthesia potentially further compromises oxygenation of the vital organs.

- Again in animals, Enflurane attenuates the sympathetic responses to haemorrhage resulting in worse haemodynamics than the non-anaesthetised state.[4]

Choice of anaesthetic agent in the shocked patient

Controlled studies on shocked patients undergoing anaesthesia are problematic due to

- differences in severity of injury or shock,
- differences in fluids administered,
- adequacy of resuscitation prior to surgery,
- haemodynamic state and degree of cardiovascular support,
- previous health most notably cardiac reserve.

Thus one must take guidance from basic anaesthetic and pharmacological principles including the principles summarised above. In addition, studies on animal models are available, case studies and series may be of interest and there are reports on the use of anaesthesia in military situations.

A major dilemma is how to provide any anaesthesia for the profoundly shocked patient. Thiopentone is said (almost certainly incorrectly) to have killed more Americans at Pearl Harbor than the Japanese! Many patients suffering from an exsanguinating injury may be so 'shocked' as to be thought to not require or be able to survive any anaesthetic administration – what used to be known as the oxygen and Pancuronium anaesthetic! While the intent to save life in this situation is laudable the absence of recordable BP does *not guarantee lack of awareness*. It is strongly recommended that, at the very least, small amounts of Midazolam are given to the patient as this will reduce the incidence of recall.[5] As the patient's condition improves, for example, as haemorrhage is controlled judicious amounts of opiods and other anaesthetic agents may be introduced.

Ketamine may be a useful option in the above circumstances but the profoundly shocked patient whose endogenous catecholamine stores have been exhausted may still suffer profound falls in BP on induction. Indeed, Ketamine has negative inotropic effects on human heart muscle *in vitro* and reduces the heart's ability to respond to β stimulation.

There are some animal studies to guide choice of anaesthesia in the shocked patient:

- Ketamine was associated with significantly increased survival compared with other agents in a model of haemorrhagic shock.[6] In that study the animals anaesthetised with Ketamine had better preservation of cell structure in the splanchnic organs.

- Ketamine was associated with increased cardiac output than Thiopentone in another animal haemorrhagic shock model.[7] Vital organ blood flow was also improved in the Ketamine group. The percentage of blood volume loss required to cause significant hypotension was significantly less in the Thiopentone group.

- In one of the few studies in high risk patients, low dose Ketamine preserved cardiac function and myocardial oxygen balance compared with Thiopentone.[8]

- In critically ill patients the use of Ketamine is more unpredictable. Most patients increase cardiac output and BP but a small percentage demonstrate falls in cardiac parameters.[9]

Choice of anaesthetic agent in the septic patient

There are no controlled studies in septic patients from the ICU undergoing surgery in the operating room. What guidance is available comes from case reports and animal studies. Total IV anaesthesia with Propofol (and more recently Remifentanil) has been poorly studied in these patients although many anaesthetists have experience of continuing Propofol sedation from ICU into theatre:

- The sympathetic stimulation associated with the use of Ketamine may result in improved haemodynamics, diuresis and reduction in the degree of cardiovascular support.[10]

- In animals with septic shock, volatile agents are associated with increases in serum lactate while Ketamine was associated with reductions in lactate. Ketamine preserved SVR and BP best.[11] To summarise a complex paper, Ketamine best preserved cardiac function and tissue oxygenation.

- In an ARDS model there is an increase in the inflammatory response and immediate mortality with volatile anaesthetic agents compared with Ketamine.[12]

Thus, animal studies and case reports strongly support the use of Ketamine in shocked and septic patients undergoing anaesthesia but caution is still advised. Unfortunately there is a shortage of convincing comparative patient studies and the above animal studies are not necessarily directly transferable into clinical practice. Most anaesthetists use the techniques they are most familiar with, either total IV anaesthesia or inhalational anaesthesia, for the critically ill patient in the operating theatre. Few have much experience of Ketamine in the UK. Therefore, despite its strong theoretical advantages it is not commonly used. Further clinical studies in this patient subgroup are urgently needed.

INTRAOPERATIVE MANAGEMENT OF HEAD INJURIES AND OTHER CAUSES OF RAISED ICP

Trauma patients frequently have concomitant head injury. The principles of anaesthesia for trauma patients with head injury are well established and covered fully in the standard anaesthesia and neuroanaesthesia texts. A recently published textbook of neuranaesthesia and critical care is listed in the suggestions for Further reading. Important principles worth emphasising include:

- Hyperventilation reduces ICP and brain volume and permits surgical access to the brain. In an ideal world hyperventilation would be monitored by jugular venous oxygen content in view of the potential for ischaemia if cerebral blood flow is reduced excessively.

- All volatile agents may increase cerebral blood flow and ICP. Hyperventilation is essential if volatile agents are used.

- Propofol infusions are increasingly popular.

- Ketamine may increase BP and ICP, and should be avoided.

- Full muscle relaxation is essential to avoid straining and coughing induced increases in ICP.

PRACTICAL CONDUCT OF ANAESTHESIA

- Conventional assessments of fitness for anaesthesia and surgery may not be helpful. The bleeding patient may not be able to be stabilised until the bleeding is controlled.

- Many of these patients require ongoing resuscitation. The **ABC** system is widely followed:

  A is airway including cervical spine protection,
  B is breathing,
  C is circulation.

  The less well-known system of **VIP** (**V**entilation, **I**nfusion and **P**erfusion) is perhaps more appropriate for surgical and trauma patients as it emphasises the interrelationship between ventilation and perfusion in overall oxygen transport and because it reminds us that the cornerstone of resuscitation in these patients is fluid infusion.

- It is an important principle that inotropes and vasopressors should not be given as a substitute for fluids in the hypovolaemic patient but perfusion of the coronary and cerebral circulations must be maintained. It is, therefore, appropriate to use such drugs to maintain perfusion of the heart and brain in the short term while one 'catches up' with blood loss.

- Critically ill patients do not always tolerate movement. Many will already be intubated. Therefore, it seems logical to transfer these patients direct to theatre rather than via the anaesthetic room. In addition, in many hospitals monitoring standards remain higher in theatre than the anaesthetic room.

- Portable monitors with full invasive monitoring facilities are commonplace and will be used for transfer of patients from ICU or A&E to theatre. It may be sensible to continue to use this monitor rather than risk confusion swapping over all the lines and cables. (Do not forget to plug in the portable monitor to maintain battery life for the journey back!)

- If invasive monitoring is not *in situ* it may be prudent (time permitting) to establish this using local anaesthesia prior to induction for beat-to-beat monitoring of this period of the anaesthetic (see below).

- Ruptured aneurysms and other cases of massive haemorrhage should be 'prepped' on the table prior to induction as discussed in the chapter on vascular anaesthesia.

- Communication and timing with theatre staff, surgeons, porters, etc. should eliminate delays in potentially difficult circumstances and environments.

INTRAOPERATIVE MONITORING

Full monitoring according to local and national protocols should be employed in all patients. In addition critically ill patients will require invasive monitoring with an indwelling arterial line for

- beat-to-beat monitoring of BP,

- sampling of blood for blood gas measurement,

- control of inotrope and vasopressor infusions;

and a central venous catheter for

- measurement of filling pressure, i.e. preload of the right ventricle (RV),

- guide to fluid requirements,

- infusion of irritant drugs, for example, inotropes, vasopressors and IV nutrition.

Central venous pressure (CVP) reflects right atrial pressure which is usually taken to reflect RV end diastolic pressure. It does *not* necessarily reflect left ventricle (LV) preload and also poorly correlates with blood volume. CVP is often used as a guide to LV function. Directional changes in CVP may reflect alterations in LV performance. However, if either ventricle becomes selectively depressed, or if there is severe pulmonary disease, changes in CVP will *not* reflect changes in LV function.

Such patients may require a pulmonary artery flotation catheter (PAFC) to enable measurements of the filling pressures at the left side of the heart (estimated by the pulmonary capillary wedge pressure, the PCWP) as the inflated balloon at the catheter tip is 'wedged' in the pulmonary artery and cardiac output and derived haemodynamic variables.

A urinary catheter is required for hourly urine volume measurement. Temperature should be monitored for all long procedures because of the dangers of perioperative hypothermia discussed above.

Monitoring strategies in the high risk surgical patient

- Invasive monitoring of elderly surgical patients has revealed a high incidence of 'hidden' abnormalities reflecting their reduced physiological reserve even in patients 'cleared' for surgery. Invasive monitoring during anaesthesia and in the postoperative period results in early recognition of problems, 'fine tuning' of cardiovascular parameters and an improved outcome.[13]

- Perioperative optimisation (discussed elsewhere) of cardiac function and oxygen transport will obviously require invasive monitoring of cardiac function – most commonly with the aid of a PAFC.

- Perioperative use of the PAFC is controversial. In the case of critically ill patients there is doubt as to the value, in terms of improved outcome, of *routine* use of the PAFC with some studies even suggesting an increased mortality associated with its use. Perioperative studies also cast doubt on the role of the PAFC in elective high risk surgery. For example, *routine* use of PAFCs during aortic surgery is not beneficial and may lead to increased complications.[14] Similarly there is no benefit from the PAFC for routine coronary artery bypass grafting (CABG) surgery.[15]

- The American Society of Anesthesiologists has published guidelines for its perioperative use[16] and there is a large multicentre trial underway in the UK which may resolve some of the controversy.

- Broad indications currently for the use of a PAFC are patients with severe disease of either ventricle, but most commonly patients with severe LV dysfunction, in order to optimise preload prior to the use of inotropes.

- In addition, the PAFC may enable early diagnosis of cardiac ischaemia if there are sudden increases in PCWP, guide haemodynamic management of septic patients and monitor pulmonary artery pressures where these are elevated.

- Paradoxically, the PAFC is not always helpful in shocked or bleeding patients in the operating theatre in whom the main aim of the anaesthetist is often to administer sufficient fluids to enable the patient to survive the necessary 'damage control' surgery – followed by fine tuning of the haemodynamic state in the ICU.

FLUID THERAPY

The crystalloid versus colloid debate

- There has been controversy over the best type of fluid for resuscitation, i.e. crystalloids or colloids. Part of the problem is the lack of studies showing a sufficiently clear superiority of one fluid type over another, sufficient to convert its opponents and without reasonable criticisms of study methodology. There are several problems with most of the available studies, for example, different species, fluids, injuries, illnesses, complications studied.

- It is not widely appreciated that many of the original US studies of crystalloids versus colloids in trauma patients were flawed. This was because most patients in both groups were given blood transfusions. In the US, patients are commonly given *whole* blood (as opposed to packed red cells in the UK), i.e. both groups received colloid from the whole blood, i.e. there was no such thing as a pure crystalloid group. Perhaps it is not surprising that few differences in outcome were detected.

- However, in most studies there is probably a skewed distribution of severity of sickness with a large group of patients who will do all right whichever fluid is given and a smaller group of patients who will die regardless of which fluid is given. These patients may mask (statistically speaking) a group of patients in whom choice of fluid may be critical. This possibility has been seized upon by the colloid enthusiasts!

There are certain statements regarding the colloid/crystalloid controversy which can be made which are reasonably accepted by both groups:

- Crystalloids replace interstitial losses. Colloids are superior at replacing plasma volume deficits – more quickly and lasting longer – giving greater increases in cardiac output and oxygen delivery. Crystalloid administration may also produce such increases but approximately three times as much will be needed with consequent delays in achieving goals of resuscitation.

- Crystalloids are cheap. Colloids are more expensive. Many centres in the US use crystalloids almost exclusively. However, it has been pointed out that whole blood may be a significant source of colloid in studies purporting to use no colloid.

- In most situations (for example routine surgery) both potentially give excellent results if appropriate amounts are used.

- Many studies show similar effects on respiratory function. Overdose of either may produce respiratory failure.

Most reasonable people do not take extreme positions in the debate. In most situations close monitoring especially with regard to fluid overload is more important than absolute choice of fluid.

However, many believe in the 'Golden Hour' for resuscitation and that, therefore, speed of resuscitation is crucial. Therefore, when restoration of blood volume, cardiac output and tissue perfusion is urgent colloids are preferable to crystalloid.

Intraoperative volume loading

In the high risk or critically ill patient generous fluid loading may be appropriate:

- Fluid loading after induction of anaesthesia to a maximum stroke volume led to a reduction of the incidence of low pHi, an index of gastric mucosal perfusion from 50% to 10%.[17]

- Intraoperative volume loading increases stroke volume and CO, resulting in a more rapid postoperative recovery and a reduced hospital stay in fractured neck of femur patients.[18]

This approach must be tempered with caution in the elderly or patients with known heart failure due to the potential risk of fluid overload precipitating pulmonary oedema. Perioperative invasive monitoring may be indicated.

However, inadequate fluid therapy is more common, more dangerous (organ hypoperfusion leading to, for example, renal failure) and less easily treated than the effects of excessive fluids which can, if necessary, be cleared with diuretic therapy.

Permissive hypovolaemia

- An important study in 1994 of penetrating trauma showed an improved survival in those patients with 'delayed' fluid resuscitation, i.e. minimal IV fluids given prior to definitive operative intervention.[19] This has been called 'permissive hypovolaemia'.

- The rationale, borne out by previous animal studies, is that full resuscitation results in

  - higher BP disrupting clot formation,

  - haemodilution and decreased viscosity disrupt clot formation,

  - dilutional coagulopathy.

- The recommendation has, therefore, been made in penetrating injury to limit fluids to maintain an MAP not > 50 until bleeding has been surgically controlled, *then* full resuscitation.

- The biggest problem is that this study was performed in *penetrating* injuries. Patients with blunt trauma (the majority) are not so likely to have definitive surgical interventions.

- This approach is also applicable in surgical cases of life-threatening haemorrhage, for example, ruptured aortic aneurysm.

Blood transfusion

From the perspective of the anaesthetist certain points are worth emphasising:

- The importance of communication with surgeon re-bleeding. On occasion the surgeon may need to be told to stop dissecting and control active bleeding to allow one to 'catch up'.

- Similarly one must communicate early with the blood bank re-requirements especially requirements for clotting factors.

- Many anaesthetists only start to consider blood transfusion once approximately 10% of the patient's blood volume (based on 80 ml/kg body weight) has been lost. With ongoing brisk haemorrhage one should not wait until 10% has been lost!

- Maintaining body temperature will minimise coagulopathy and blood loss as previously described.

- Maintaining blood volume is probably more important in the short term than maintaining Hb. However, with major haemorrhage blood *will* be needed!

- Autologous transfusion systems, for example, 'cell savers' should be considered for appropriate 'clean' operations.

INOTROPES AND VASOACTIVE DRUGS

In addition to the normal anaesthetic goals that pertain to all patients one must pay special interest to the maintenance of organ blood flow and function in the critically ill patient. This is obviously the case for all our patients but fortunately the vast majority of low risk patients present few problems and rarely need any form of circulatory support. In septic or shocked patients this is the norm and the choice of inotropes and vasopressors and monitoring of the circulation are discussed below:

- Adequate filling pressures and intravascular volume are crucial prior to anaesthesia and also the use of inotropic agents. With hypovolaemia the vasodilator effects of inotropic agents such as Dobutamine predominate leading to hypotension. The use of vasopressors in hypovolaemia will reduce splanchnic and muscle blood flow. Indeed, the use of noradrenaline in haemorrhagic shock is a useful animal model of acute tubular necrosis!

- Cardiac function can be severely compromised in haemorrhagic shock so that an element of cardiogenic shock contributes to the shocked state. In such cases the response to resuscitation may be compromised and invasive monitoring and/or inotropes required as detailed below. As early as the 1950s the contribution of the heart to progressive, irreversible shock was recognised and it was also demonstrated that the homeostatic mechanisms and vasoconstriction were not sufficient to maintain coronary perfusion in severe haemorrhage. Therefore, cardiac dysfunction needs to be detected and corrected as early after injury as possible.

- For myocardial support in the failing heart and low output states Dobutamine is probably the agent of choice.

- For vascular support, for example, with abnormal vasodilation, noradrenaline is probably the agent of choice.

- In view of concerns relating to gut blood flow and lactic acidosis the role of adrenaline infusions perioperatively is controversial.

- For information on the support of regional circulations including the use of Dopamine and Dopexamine the chapters on Perioperative Optimisation and Renal Insufficiency should be consulted.

Many critically ill patients in the operating theatre will have severe sepsis. The latest international guidelines on management of septic shock support the use of noradrenaline as first line agent in septic shock once volume resuscitation has been achieved.[20] The two main arguments against the use of noradrenaline, i.e.

- reduced renal blood flow,

- reduced cardiac output secondary to vasoconstriction induced increases in afterload

are unfounded. In fact, in septic shock noradrenaline improves urine volumes and creatinine clearance[21] and improves cardiac output.[22]

The possibility of altered organ blood flow intraoperatively due to interactions between anaesthetic agents and vasoactive drugs is poorly understood.

OXYGEN TRANSPORT IN THE HIGH RISK OR CRITICALLY ILL SURGICAL PATIENT

Differences between haemorrhagic shock and traumatic shock

Haemorrhage results in well-known physiologic changes. Traumatic shock includes these responses but they are modified by the tissue injury and its associated inflammatory response. This has several practical effects:

- HR responds to haemorrhage by an initial tachycardia followed eventually by a progressive bradycardia. This has been labelled as a 'paradoxical bradycardia' but there is nothing paradoxical about the heart slowing in the absence of adequate venous return in an attempt to maintain stroke volume. This *is* seen following, for example, ruptured ectopic pregnancy. With tissue injury there is no late slowing of the heart and tachycardia continues.

- BP is maintained by vasoconstriction until more than one-third of blood volume has been lost. With tissue injury, BP is maintained to a greater degree by the surge in catecholamines and other nociceptive stimuli but this is at the expense of tissue perfusion due to excessive vasoconstriction.

- Animal studies show that for an equivalent degree of blood loss, traumatic injury results in greater tissue hypoperfusion and a greater 'injury' than simple haemorrhage.

- The wound and fracture sites are metabolically active with a resultant requirement for increased oxygen consumption and glucose oxidation – the concept of 'the wound as an organ'. In addition to the local reasons for increased metabolic demands, there are systemic inflammatory and catabolic causes of increased metabolic demand requiring an increased cardiac output compared to normal. This may imply a need for increased cardiac output and oxygen delivery in trauma and high risk surgical patients – Shoemaker's optimal goals as discussed in the chapter on Perioperative Optimisation.

Optimal goals

The best evidence for a beneficial therapeutic effect of maximising oxygen transport according to previously identified optimal goals is from studies where therapy was initiated very early in the presence of tissue hypoperfusion, i.e. preoperatively in high risk surgical patients. Shoemaker's original prospective, randomised study demonstrating the virtues of optimising oxygen transport was performed in surgical patients.[23]

A thought provoking review[24] points out that there are conflicting priorities in managing surgical patients at risk of myocardial ischaemia, for example, using β blockers and those in whom the cardiac output and oxygen delivery need to be increased, for example, using inotropes. Both groups are at risk of an adverse outcome but the approach is different and identification of the group that patients belong to is important. These issues are further explored in the chapter on Perioperative Optimisation.

Oxygen debt and lactic acidosis in the high risk surgical patient

Even when oxygen delivery is well maintained oxygen consumption falls under anaesthesia. Animal studies show that anaesthesia reduces tissue oxygen extraction especially in septic models. This occurs with all agents but is associated with lactic acidosis only with volatile agents. Ketamine may increase oxygen extraction by the tissues compared with volatile and IV barbiturate techniques.[25]

Thus, although anaesthesia reduces metabolic rate and oxygen demand this may be countered in the critically ill patient by the reduction in the tissue's ability to extract oxygen. An oxygen debt may develop especially if there are falls in cardiac output and/or oxygen delivery below a critical level.[26] Worryingly, the reduction of tissue oxygen extraction under anaesthesia may increase the threshold for oxygen delivery to be 'critical',[27] i.e. lesser degrees of fall in cardiac output and oxygen delivery may result in tissue hypoxia under anaesthesia.

This has obvious implications for anaesthesia of the critically ill or shocked patient, in whom maintenance of cardiac output and oxygen delivery are crucial.

There are many studies demonstrating that high risk surgical patients develop an intraoperative 'oxygen debt', the magnitude and duration of which correlates with the development of lactic acidosis, organ failure and increased mortality.[28–30] This oxygen debt is postulated to potentially arise from anaesthetic cardiac depression, direct anaesthetic reductions in tissue oxygen uptake as already described, failure to maintain adequate fluid intake during surgery and perhaps hypothermia.

The crucial message is that high risk surgical patients may have reduced cardiac reserves, especially in the elderly, suffer occult tissue hypoperfusion with a developing oxygen debt postoperatively, proceed to multiple organ failure if there is no intervention to reverse the tissue hypoperfusion and have a higher mortality than patients who *do* have sufficient reserves to reverse their oxygen debt and prevent serious tissue hypoxia. Appropriate interventions may include fluid therapy, oxygen, inotropes and vasopressors.

However, recent studies suggest that not all metabolic acidosis under anaesthesia is due to oxygen debt and/or lactic acidosis. Rapid infusion of 0.9% saline can cause significant hyperchloraemic metabolic acidosis.[31,32] The common treatment of administering more fluid for intraoperative acidosis may be inappropriate if the fluid administered has a high chloride content such as saline or Gelofusine. Measurement of serum lactate and chloride may be helpful in distinguishing the cause of the intraoperative acidosis.

Further reading

Intensive Care Society. *Guidelines for Transport of the Critically Ill Adult*, 1997.

The Association of Anaesthetists of Great Britain and Ireland and The Neuroanaesthesia Society of Great Britain and Ireland. *Recommendations for the Transfer of Patients with Acute Head Injuries to Neurosurgical Units*, 1996.

Grande CM. *Textbook of Trauma Anesthesia and Critical Care*, 1993. St Louis: Mosby.

Matta BF, Menon DK, Turner JM (eds). *Textbook of Neuroanaesthesia and Critical Care*, 2000. London: Greenwich Medical Media.

References

1. Schmied H, Kurz A, Sessler DI, Kozek S, Reiter A. Mild hypothermia increases blood loss and transfusion requirements during total hip arthroplasty. *Lancet* 1996; **347**: 289–92.

2. Frank SM, Fleisher LA, Breslow MJ, Higgins MS, Olson KF *et al.* Perioperative maintenance of normothermia reduces the incidence of morbid cardiac events: a randomised clinical trial. *JAMA* 1997; **227**: 1127–43.

3. Durieux ME, Sperry RJ, Longnecker DE. Effects of hypoxemia on regional blood flows during anesthesia with halothane, enflurane, or isoflurane. *Anesthesiology* 1992; **76**: 402–8.

4. Mayer N, Zimpler M, Kotai E *et al*. Enflurane alters compensatory hemodynamic and humoral responses to hemorrhage. *Circ Shock* 1990; **30**: 165–70.

5. Bogetz MS, Katz JA. Recall of surgery for major trauma. *Anesthesiology* 1984; **61**: 6–9.

6. Longnecker DE, Sturgill BC. Influence of anesthetic agent on survival following hemorrhage. *Anaesthesiology* 1976; **45**: 516–21.

7. Idvall J. Influence of ketamine anesthesia on cardiac output and tissue perfusion in rats subjected to hemorrhage. *Anesthesiology* 1981; **55**: 297–304.

8. Pedersen T, Engback J, Klausen NO *et al*. Effects of low dose ketamine and thiopentone on cardiac performance and myocardial oxygen balance in high risk patients. *Acta Anaesthesiol Scand* 1982; **26**: 235–9.

9. Lippmann M, Appel PL, Mok MS *et al*. Sequential cardiorespiratory patterns of anesthetic induction with ketamine in critically ill patients. *Crit Care Med* 1983; **11**: 730–4.

10. Yli-Hankala A, Kirvela M, Randell T *et al*. Ketamine anaesthesia in a patient with septic shock. *Acta Anaesthesiol Scand* 1992; **36**: 483–5.

11. Van der Linden P, Gilbart E, Engelman E *et al*. Comparison of halothane, isoflurane, alfentanil and ketamine in experimental septic shock. *Anesth Analg* 1990; **70**: 608–17.

12. Nader-Djalal N, Knight PR, Bacon MF *et al*. Alterations in the course of acid-induced lung injury in rats after general anesthesia: volatile anesthetics versus ketamine. *Anesth Analg* 1998; **86**: 141–6.

13. Del Guercio LRN, Cohn JD. Monitoring operative risk in the elderly. *JAMA* 1980; **297**: 845–50.

14. Valentine RJ, Duke ML, Inman MH *et al*. Effectiveness of pulmonary artery catheters in aortic surgery: a randomized trial. *J Vasc Surg* 1998; **27**: 203–11.

15. Tuman KJ, McCarthy RJ, Spiess BD *et al*. Effect of pulmonary artery catheterization on outcome in patients undergoing coronary artery surgery. *Anesthesiology* 1989; **70**: 199–206.

16. Practice guidelines for pulmonary artery catheterization. A report by the American Society of Anesthesiologists Task Force on Pulmonary Artery Catheterization. *Anesthesiology* 1993; **78**: 380–94.

17. Mythen MG, Webb AR. Perioperative plasma volume expansion reduces the incidence of gut mucosal hypoperfusion during cardiac surgery. *Arch Surg* 1995; **130**: 423–9.

18. Sinclair S, James S, Singer M. Intraoperative intravascular volume optimisation and length of hospital stay after repair of proximal femoral fracture: randomised controlled trial. *Br Med J* 1997; **315**: 909–12.

19. Bickell WH, Wall MJ Jr, Pepe PE, Martin RR, Ginger VF *et al.* Immediate versus delayed fluid resuscitation for hypotensive patients with penetrating torso injuries. *N Engl J Med* 1994; **331**: 1105–9.

20. Vincent JL. Hemodynamic support in septic shock. *Inten Care Med* 2001; **27**: S80–92.

21. Redl-Wenzl EM, Armbruster C, Edelmann G, Fischl E, Kolacny M *et al.* The effects of norepinephrine on hemodynamics and renal function in severe septic shock states. *Inten Care Med* 1993; **19**: 151–4.

22. Martin C, Viviand X, Arnaud S *et al.* Effects of norepinephrine plus dobutamine or norepinephrine alone on left ventricular performance of septic shock patients. *Crit Care Med* 1999; **7**: 1708–13.

23. Shoemaker WC, Appel PL, Kram HB, Waxman K, Lee TS. Prospective trial of supranormal values of survivors as therapeutic goals in high-risk surgical patients. *Chest* 1988; **94**: 1176–86.

24. Juste RN, Lawson AD, Soni N. Minimising cardiac anaesthetic risk: the tortoise or the hare? *Anaesthesia* 1996; **51**: 255–62.

25. Van der Linden P, Gilbart E, Engelman E *et al.* Effects of anesthetic agents on systemic critical O_2 delivery. *J Appl Physiol* 1991; **71**: 83–93.

26. Lugo G, Arizpe D, Dominguez G. Relationship between oxygen consumption and oxygen delivery during anesthesia in high-risk surgical patients. *Crit Care Med* 1993; **21**: 64–9.

27. Van der Linden P, Schmartz D, Gilbart E *et al.* Effects of propofol, etomidate, and pentobarbital on critical oxygen delivery. *Crit Care Med* 2000; **28**: 2492–9.

28. Shoemaker WC, Appel PL, Kram HB. Role of oxygen debt in the development of organ failure sepsis, and death in high-risk surgical patients. *Chest* 1992; **102**: 208–15.

29. Shoemaker WC, Appel PL, Kram HB. Tissue oxygen debt as a determinant of lethal and nonlethal postoperative organ failure. *Crit Care Med* 1988; **16**: 1118–20.

30. Hess W, Frank C, Hornburg B. Prolonged oxygen debt after abdominal aortic surgery. *J Cardiothorac Vasc Anesth* 1997; **11**: 149–54.

31. Scheingraber S, Rehm M, Sehmisch C *et al.* Rapid saline infusion produces hyperchloremic acidosis in patients undergoing gynecologic surgery. *Anesthesiology* 1999; **90**: 1265–70.

32. Waters JH, Miller LR, Clack S *et al.* Cause of metabolic acidosis in prolonged surgery. *Crit Care Med* 1999; **27**: 2142–6.

7

THE ELDERLY PATIENT

Data from the Office for National Statistics[1] showed that, in 1997, the average life expectancy for a man was 74 years and for a woman 79 years. The mid-1999 population demographics revealed that 9.8 million (16.5%) of the population of the United Kingdom were over pensionable age and that was expected to rise by another 4.6 million by the year 2023:

- With the advancement of anaesthetic and surgical techniques, more and more elderly patients are presenting for major elective and emergency surgery.

- It is vital therefore that the practising anaesthetist is aware of the important differences that exist between the elderly patient and the young adult.

Ageing is a continuous process once the organism has reached maturity. There is no strict, defined age when an adult becomes elderly. In this chapter, like other texts, the elderly patient will be assumed to be aged 65 years or over.

PHYSIOLOGICAL CHANGES ASSOCIATED WITH AGEING

After the age of 30 years there is a gradual deterioration in organ function. The rate and extent of decline often determines those who are 'physiologically young for their age' or those who are 'physiologically old for their age'.

The ageing cardiovascular system[2–6]

Most of the investigation of the cardiovascular system in human adults comes from longitudinal studies of cohorts of adults as they age and in aged individuals with no heart disease. Most investigation has been with echocardiography or angiographic or radionuclide imaging of the heart. Whether the changes in the vascular system lead to compensatory changes in the heart or whether both occur simultaneously and independently is a matter of debate:

- The arterial system becomes less compliant due to a loss in elastic tissue in the vessel wall. This results in an increased left ventricular afterload and systolic hypertension. The arteries also become less responsive to vasodilators such as nitric oxide, atrial naturetic peptide and β_2 adreno-ceptor stimulation.

- The venous system also becomes less compliant with a reduction in the strength of smooth muscle contraction within the vessel wall. The elderly therefore have less blood in the capacitance vessels and less ability to squeeze this blood into the central circulation in the face of intravascular fluid depletion.

- The ventricle hypertrophies with age. This may be in part as a response to the increased afterload and as a primary effect of ageing. Ventricular hypertrophy reduces ventricular compliance, increases left ventricular end diastolic pressure (LVEDP) and reduces early diastolic filling of the ventricle. The elevated LVEDP increases the importance of atrial contraction (hence sinus rhythm) on late ventricular filling. Atrial hyper-trophy develops to the increased impedance (LVEDP) to atrial emptying.

- The myocardium and pacemaker cells become less responsive to β_2 adrenoceptor stimulation. Therefore there is a reduction in both inotropic and chronotropic effects of β_2 stimulation.

- At rest cardiac index is unchanged or reduced in proportion to the reduction in basal metabolic rate or silent coronary artery disease. The situation during exercise is markedly different to the young adult. In the exercising young adult, cardiac output is increased by an increased heart rate and ejection fraction (i.e. a lower left ventricular end diastolic and systolic volume (LVEDV and LVESV)). In the elderly, heart rate **falls** during exercise, LVEDV **increases** (by 20–30%) but LVESV decreases less, and therefore ejection fraction increases less, than in the young adult. It is apparent then, that cardiac output in the elderly patient is more pre-load dependent than in the young adult during times of cardiovascular stress.

- Pacemaker activity of the heart declines with age. The cells of the sino-atrial (SA) node atrophy, conduction through the atrioventricular (AV) node is increased and conduction through the bundles is impaired. Heart block, bundle branch block and arrhythmias (both brady- and tachyarrythmias) become increasingly common with age.

- Coronary artery vascular resistance increases in the elderly because of the increased LVEDP and ventricular hypertrophy, but the reduced coronary flow is counterbalanced by a reduced myocardial oxygen consumption.

Ageing of the respiratory system[7-9]

As one ages there are changes in the structure of the lung and airways along with changes in the thoracic wall. These fundamental structural changes lead to the physiological changes seen with advancing age:

- There is a loss in elastic tissue within the lung parenchyma as well as loss of alveolar surface area and therefore loss in surface tension forces. Both elastic tissue and surface tension contribute to the elastic recoil of the lung, hence the compliance of the ageing lung is **increased** (compliance being the reciprocal of elastance). Calcification of the costal cartilage and the rib articulations reduce the thoracic compliance that counterbalances the increased lung compliance. There is some debate as to whether total compliance is unaltered or reduced because of the greater reduction in thoracic compliance over the increase in lung compliance.

- The losses in alveolar surface area results in V/Q mismatch, an increased physiological shunt (increased A-a gradient) and consequently a lower PaO_2. The PaO_2 can be estimated from the formula: PaO_2 (mmHg) = $100 - Age/3$.

- Changes in lung volumes also contribute to an increased physiological shunt. Throughout life, there is an increase in the volume of air required to prevent small airway collapse also known as closing volume (CV). At around 45 years of age, CV exceeds functional residual capacity (FRC) in the supine position and in the seated position by 65 years of age. Once CV exceeds FRC then airway closure occurs during tidal ventilation. The increase in CV can, on the whole, be explained by the loss in elastic tissue with age.

- Aside from an increase in CV with age there is an increase in residual volume. FRC, the point at which the outward pull of the thorax is balanced by the tendency for the lung to collapse, is unchanged at the expense of a reduced expiratory reserve volume (ERV). As ERV is reduced it follows that vital capacity (VC) must be reduced. It is believed that total lung capacity is unchanged, or only reduced slightly (10%) with age.

- The large airways increase in size as one ages resulting in an increased anatomical and physiological deadspace. Airway resistance is unchanged as the resistance (proximal) airways dilate and the smaller, distal, airways collapse thus offsetting each other. Although total compliance is unchanged or marginally reduced, the loss in elasticity of the lungs and rigidity of the chest wall increases the work of breathing.

- The elderly have a diminished response to both hypercapnia and hypoxia. The elderly, like the younger adult are able to increase respiratory rate but are unable to increase tidal volume in response to an abnormal PaO_2 or $PaCO_2$. The reason for the fall in tidal volume is postulated to be a reduced sensitivity or a reduced output from the respiratory centre rather than a loss in respiratory muscle power with age.

- The elderly have blunted protective laryngeal reflexes and therefore are more at risk of pulmonary aspiration during anaesthesia.

- Pulmonary vascular resistance increases with age but it is doubtful if this is of any clinical significance.

Changes in renal function with age[10,11]

Data regarding the changes in the kidney with age is primarily from cross-sectional studies and histological findings. Some data is available from longitudinal studies and tends to be more reliable than the former sources because it excludes renal dysfunction as a result of age related changes.

- Renal mass declines with age. After the 3rd decade there is 1% loss per year. The reduction in mass is due to glomerular loss (up to 30% by the 8th decade) which is predominantly cortical. The exact cause of the glomerular atrophy is unknown but it mirrors a reduction in renal blood and plasma flow (10% per decade).

- Loss of glomeruli has been implicated in the fall in glomerular filtration rate (GFR) with age. Absolute creatinine clearance falls approximately $1 \, ml/min/1.73 \, m^2$ per year, or from $140 \, ml/min/1.73 \, m^2$ in the 3rd decade to $97 \, ml/min/1.73 \, m^2$ in the 8th decade. However, plasma creatinine levels are unchanged in the elderly because a reduced muscle mass results in a reduced production of creatinine.

- Renal tubular function declines with age. Inulin clearance, which represents tubular secretory function declines and is paralleled by deterioration in reabsorptive function. Tubular dysfunction may be explained by the loss of glomerular units and a reduction in metabolically active tubular cells with age.

- The aged kidney is less effective at concentrating urine and conserving water in the face of water deprivation. This may result from a lowering in the medullary concentration gradient caused by a disturbance of the counter-current mechanism due to alterations in renal blood flow and a relative resistance to anti–diuretic hormone (ADH). Moreover thirst perception during periods of dehydration is impaired. The nephron is also impaired in its ability to dilute the urine in the face of water overload.

- The elderly face problems in salt conservation. Plasma renin and aldosterone levels are reduced in the elderly. This may be due to the relative unresponsiveness to β_2 receptor stimulation as renin is released in response to β_2 adrenoceptor stimulation. Moreover, changes in the heart with age lead to atrial distension and release of atrial natriuretic factor (ANF) which also suppresses renin and aldosterone release. Not only does the relative deficiency of these two hormones lead to sodium loss but it places the elderly at risk of hyperkalaemia.

The effect of age on hepatic function[12,13]

The liver, like most other organs, involutes with age, so by the 8th decade the liver has lost two-fifths of its mass. There is also a reduction in hepatic blood flow that not only reflects the loss in hepatic cellular mass but also an absolute reduction in terms of percentage of cardiac output. Despite the reduction in mass and blood flow, it appears that hepatocellular enzyme function is preserved with advancing age. *In vitro* studies in patients with normal histology on liver biopsy failed to demonstrate any deterioration in hepatic microsomal oxygenase or hydrolase activity (phase I metabolic reactions) and also showed that reduced glutathione (phase II conjugation reactions and a major hepatic anti-oxidant) concentrations are maintained.

In parallel with the apparent preservation of hepatocellular function, serum concentration of bilirubin, alkaline phosphatase, and transaminases are unaffected by age. Coagulation studies are also unchanged by age but there is a gradual decline in serum albumin concentration.

Changes in the nervous system with age[14,15]

Memory loss, confusion and dementia are the clinical manifestations of ageing of the brain. Unlike other organs there are no readily applicable tests of 'brain function' but the following are generally accepted as age related changes, with or without clinical manifestation:

- Normal pressure hydrocephalus results from global atrophy of the brain and an increase in cerebrospinal fluid (CSF) volume. The brain weighs 20% less by the 8th decade than in the 2nd decade of life and CSF volume increases by 10% in the same time period.

- Cerebral blood flow is reduced in line with brain volume but auto-regulation to carbon dioxide and mean arterial blood pressure is preserved.

- Within the brain the most metabolically active cells (grey matter of the cerebral and cerebellar cortices, basal ganglia, thalamus) atrophy more than the white matter. Regional blood flow reflects the neuronal loss with flow to the grey matter reduced more than that to the white.

- The levels of excitatory neurotransmitters (norepinephrine, serotonin, dopamine and tryrosine) are reduced.

The peripheral neurones like their counterparts in the brain undergo age related degeneration. In particular there is:

- An increased threshold to stimulate sensory organs, such as pain corpuscles, and a reduced conduction velocity in afferent neurones and ascending spinocortical tracts. There is also a reduced conduction velocity in motor neurones and in the corticospinal tracts so that the reflex arc for painful stimuli is increased and righting reflexes are impaired.

- Skeletal muscle mass is reduced and extrajunctional acetylcholine receptors increase in response to degeneration of motor neurones.

Neuroendocrine changes with age[16]

Ageing produces a state akin to a hyperadrenergic state. The impaired responses in the elderly to β_2 adrenoceptor stimulation leads to increased plasma norepinephrine and epinephrine concentrations (2–4-fold) despite atrophy of the adrenal medulla. Cardiovascular reflexes are also impaired in the elderly. Reduced responsiveness of the baroreceptors results in an underdamped cardiovascular system and there is a reduced vasoconstrictor response to cold with less heart rate change in response to changes in posture. The elderly are therefore more vulnerable to cardiovascular instability, particularly during sympathetic blockade.

Changes in body fluid composition and metabolism with ageing

The key changes that occur are summarised below:

- Basal metabolic rate falls as a consequence of a reduced skeletal mass and a reduction in the metabolically active areas of the brain, kidney and liver.

- Increased body fat results in a reduction in total body water.

- Testosterone and tri-iodothyronine levels are reduced.

- Glucose intolerance occurs.

CHANGES IN PHARMACOKINETICS AND PHARMACODYNAMICS WITH AGE[17,18]

In general absorption of drugs from the gastrointestinal tract is unaffected by age. There are, however, important changes in distribution, metabolism and elimination of drugs because of age related changes of the organs.

- A reduction in total body water means that the volume of distribution of water soluble drugs (e.g. non-depolarising muscle relaxants) is decreased with an effective increase in the tissue concentration. Conversely, an increase in body fat results in an increased volume of distribution for lipid soluble drugs.

- The reduction in albumin concentration in the elderly increases the free fraction of protein bound (i.e. lipid soluble) drugs and therefore increases the bioavailabilty at their effector sites.

- Hepatic clearance of a drug is dependent on three factors, the intrinsic clearance (CL_{int}), the free fraction of the drug (f) and the hepatic blood flow (Q_H). The hepatic clearance of drugs with a low CL_{int} is dependent on CL_{int} and f and are said to be 'capacity limited'. Examples of such drugs are barbiturates, benzodiazepines and theophyllines. If the free fraction of a highly protein bound drug is increased, then the hepatic clearance becomes more dependent upon Q_H than CL_{int}. The elderly have a reduced Q_H but CL_{int} is largely unchanged. Therefore the hepatic clearance of capacity limited drugs with low protein binding is unchanged with age. The reduction in serum albumin will increase f of highly protein bound drugs (e.g. thiopentone) and so their hepatic clearance will be reduced as a result of a reduced Q_H.

- Drugs with a high CL_{int} will be dependent on Q_H only for the hepatic clearance. They are said to be 'flow limited' and their clearance will be reduced as a result in the age related fall in Q_H. Examples of flow limited drugs are β-blockers, tricyclic anti-depressants, opioid analgesics and amide local anaesthetics.

- Biliary excretion of drug metabolites is unaffected by age, but renal excretion of water soluble drugs and drug metabolites may be reduced by age related reduction in GFR and tubular secretion.

- As well as changes in drug pharmacokinetics (e.g. increased free fraction of drugs, reduced volume of distribution, reduced clearance) the increased sensitivity to some drugs in the elderly is also due to pharmacodynamic changes. The reduction in excitatory neurotransmitters in the brain with grey matter atrophy is thought to be the basis for the enhanced sensitivity to intravenous induction agents and reduced

MAC to volatile anaesthetics. Changes in receptor sensitivity may also account for the enhanced analgesia seen with morphine, and altered sensitivity to benzodiazepines.

CO-EXISTING DISEASE AND AGE RELATED ORGAN DYSFUNCTION

The deterioration in the various organ systems described above can be accelerated and worsened by co-existing disease. These diseases are more likely to be encountered with advancing age:

- Hypertension, (essential or secondary to other diseases), diabetes mellitus, smoking and hyperlipidaemia all predispose to atheromatous disease of the arteries. This may present as angina or myocardial infarction, cerebrovascular disease, peripheral vascular insufficiency and abdominal aneurysm formation.

- Cardiac function may also be worsened by valvular abnormalities. Rheumatic fever, age related fibrosis and calcification can lead to stenotic valves, whilst ischaemic heart disease, rheumatoid arthritis (RA), connective tissue diseases (CTD), hypertension and even stenotic valves (aortic) may result in regurgitant valves.

- Pulmonary function is particularly affected by smoking and can result in emphysema or chronic bronchitis. Chronic asthma may also lead to fixed obstructive airways disease.

- Glomerulonephritis, hypertension, diabetes mellitus, RA, CTD and atheroma of the abdominal aorta and/or renal arteries can cause premature renal failure. It should be remembered that renal failure is an important cause of hypertension.

- Chronic alcohol ingestion is the major cause of cirrhosis and hepatocellular failure and may be associated with a dilated cardiomyopathy. Other rarer causes of liver dysfunction are primary biliary cirrhosis, chronic active hepatitis (post viral or autoimmune), α_1 antitrypsin deficiency (associated with emphysema) and drug therapy.

- It is important not to forget that drug therapy for medical conditions may adversely affect some organs. Examples would include renal damage from use of non-steroidal anti-inflammatory agents and penicillamine used in the treatment of RA. The liver particularly can be adversely affected by a long list of drugs and this should be borne in mind if faced with abnormal liver function tests or jaundice.

- Acute confusional states in the elderly may also be drug induced and usually resolve once the drug is discontinued.

ANAESTHESIA FOR THE ELDERLY PATIENT

The two recent CEPOD reports[19,20] highlighted the impact that the elderly have upon anaesthetic and surgical specialties:

- The 2000 report showed that the number of elderly patients (over 60 years for females and over 65 for males) presenting for surgery had increased from the 1990 report.

- In 1998/99, over 90% of patients were aged 60 years or more, with 38% over 80 years of age.

- Only 35% of procedures were deemed to be elective or scheduled, whilst 50% were urgent and the remainder emergency procedures.

- The majority of the elderly patients presented for general (42%), orthopaedic (22%) or vascular procedures (14%) and 84% were deemed by the anaesthetist to be of ASA 3 or more.

One of the key points in the 2000 report was that:

- 'The profile of patients who die within 30 days of an operation has changed since the report of 1990. Patients are more likely to be older, have undergone an urgent operation, be of poorer physical status and have co-existing cardiovascular or neurological disorder'.

The 1999 CEPOD report that looked specifically at patients over 90 years at the time of operation recognised that 'elderly patients have a high incidence of co-existing disorders and a high risk of early post-operative death'.

Pre-operative preparation

The pre-operative visit is essential for:

- initiating the patient – anaesthetist relationship and helping allay anxiety,

- determining the presence of co-existing diseases,

- planning any pre-operative investigations,

- choice of anaesthetic technique,

- method of post-operative analgesia,

- determining post-operative placement (ward, high depency unit (HDU), intensive care unit (ICU)).

The pre-operative visit for the elderly is often more taxing and takes longer than in the younger adult. Elderly patients may have cognitive impairment, memory loss and impaired hearing and vision. Moreover they might not understand what an anaesthetist is or does! Extraction of information can be prolonged and difficult, so it is vital that the patient's notes be available for perusal.

The elderly patient should have the same assessment as a younger patient, but with particular emphasis on

- A functional assessment of their cardiorespiratory status. It is important to realise that the elderly often have different symptoms of a disease. For example, ischaemic heart disease will often present as dyspnoea rather than chest pain. The reason can be explained on the basis of the age related cardiac changes, in that myocardial ischaemia further elevates the LVEDP and results in pulmonary oedema. In general a person able to climb a flight of stairs or walk up a gentle hill has a lower post-operative cardiac mortality than one who is housebound by their symptoms.

- Assessment of hydration is important but also difficult. As emphasised before, the elderly are prone to dehydration during times of fasting and hypovolaemia worsens cardiac performance and increases post-operative complications. The signs of dehydration such as loss of skin turgor, dry eyes and mouth are common findings in the elderly so one will have to look for more subtle signs such as loss of jugular venous pulsation in the supine position, postural hypotension and a raised urea. Fluid balance charts should be consulted to help with assessment of fluid status. Dehydration should be corrected pre-operatively with the use of central venous pressure monitoring as necessary to prevent tipping the patient into pulmonary oedema.

- The presence of cardiac murmurs, particularly of the aortic valve, should be sought, especially if a regional anaesthetic technique is being considered.

- The history and examination of the patient largely determines pre-operative investigations. It is generally agreed that all patients over 65 years of age should have a full blood count, urea and electrolytes and an ECG. One must realise that these investigations may show no abnormality despite the presence of age related organ dysfunction. When ordering more advanced investigations one should give thought to the accuracy of the results. For example, an exercise ECG may be of limited value when the patient is disabled by arthritis so radionuclide imaging or stress echocardiography of the heart may be more appropriate.

- Elderly patients should not be denied premedication but the drugs prescribed should be done so with knowledge of the altered pharmacokinetics and dynamics in the elderly.

- The age, physical status of the patient, the degree of urgency and the type of surgery performed determine post-operative outcome. Therefore very careful consideration should be given to the risk–benefit when an elderly patient of poor physical status presents for major surgery. Where risks outweigh perceived benefit then surgery should be deferred.

Anaesthetic technique

The overriding goal of the anaesthetist is to maintain global oxygen delivery to the patient. In effect this means:

- avoidance of hypotension/hypovolaemia,

- avoidance of hypoxia,

- avoidance of anaemia,

- these principles must be adhered to in elderly patients along with the avoidance of hypothermia.

Specific problems that can be encountered during anaesthesia for the elderly are:

- The elderly often have fragile veins making venous access difficult.

- Elderly patients have thin skin and arthritic joints. Special care should be taken when transferring and positioning on the operating table. All bony prominences should be well padded.

- Elderly patients are more at risk of hypothermia both during general anaesthesia (GA) and regional anaesthesia.[21,22] Warming mattresses, warmed intravenous fluids and warm air blowers must be readily available and used for all but the shortest of cases.

- The 1999 CEPOD report[19] highlighted the high incidence of intra-operative hypotension and how this was largely inadequately treated. In major surgical cases or cases in which there is expected to be large fluid losses, invasive monitoring of blood pressure and central venous pressure should be instituted. There should be earlier use of inotropic cardio-vascular support when hypotension fails to respond to fluid loading.

The choice of anaesthetic technique depends on the type of surgery proposed, the physical status of the patient and patient preference. A recent meta-analysis suggests that regional techniques alone or combined with GA significantly reduces post-operative morbidity.[23] A regional technique should be considered for limb, perineum and lower abdominal surgery and for laparotomy when combined with GA.

When choosing GA in the elderly, the following should be considered:

- Edentulous patients may present a difficult airway once anaesthesia is induced as the face 'collapses' making a seal with the facemask, and therefore ventilation difficult. Cervical spondylosis may make intubation difficult as neck extension is reduced.

- All elderly patients should be preoxygenated prior to induction of anaesthesia. Intravenous induction agents should be given slowly. In general the induction dose is lower and induction time prolonged. The MAC of inhalational agents is reduced but the dose of both depolarising and non-depolarising muscle relaxants is the same as a younger adult.

- The elderly are more sensitive to opioid analgesics but have delayed elimination and so doses should be reduced and dosing interval prolonged.

- Inhalational anaesthetic agents all depress the ventilatory responses to hypoxia and hypercarbia and this will be exacerbated in the elderly who already have blunted responses to changes in oxygen and carbon dioxide levels. All elderly patients should receive supplementary oxygen in the recovery room and probably continued on the ward.

Regional anaesthesia (spinal subarachnoid block and epidural) can be used alone or in conjunction with GA. It is the author's belief that spinal blockade should be used alone and that only epidural blockade is combined with GA. Points to consider in the elderly for regional anaesthesia are:

- Informed consent must be obtained from the patient. The only exception to this is where the patients cannot give consent (e.g. senile dementia) and it is felt that a regional technique is in the best interests of the patient (e.g. fractured neck of femur).

- Conditions that lead to a fixed cardiac output (e.g. aortic stenosis) and significant coagulopathy are excluded. A number of elderly patients are on low dose aspirin (<300 mg) and this is generally deemed not to be a contraindication to regional anaesthesia.[24]

- Regional anaesthesia may be more technically difficult in the elderly due to osteoarthritis, kyphoscoliosis and osteoporotic collapse. Vertebral collapse means that the spinal cord ends at a lower vertebral level in the elderly and is at risk of damage if the L3/4 space is used. A recent study has shown that there is a great variability between the surface localisation of the L3/4 space and the true space[25] and a case report has highlighted the risk to the spinal cord when the wrong interspace is identified.[26]

- Sympathetic blockade reduces cardiac preload and in the elderly may result in profound hypotension which must be treated promptly and aggressively with fluids and vasoconstrictors.

Post-operative care

Post-operative care for any patient involves four basic principles, namely the post-operative visit, post-operative analgesic regimen, fluid and oxygen therapy and post-operative placement of the patient.

- The post-operative visit is important to the anaesthetist and the patient. It should be performed on everyone and be viewed as the opportunity to review the patient and check that post-operative instructions have been followed. If the patient is not progressing as well as expected it affords time to institute more aggressive management and perhaps transfer to a higher dependency level.

- Fluid prescription post-operatively will depend upon the nature of the procedure performed, the expected ongoing losses and the expected period that oral intake will be limited. Any prescription must take into account the volume of ongoing loss as well as the daily maintenance requirements. A well organised fluid balance chart is invaluable. Ongoing losses that are extracellular should be replaced with a balanced salt solution such as compound sodium lactate. Maintenance fluids can be roughly calculated from 60 ml/hr for the first 30 kg body weight plus 1 ml/hr for each kg thereafter and should total 1 mmol/kg of Na^+ and K^+ every 24 h.

- Oxygen prescription also depends on the nature of the procedure and the pre-existing medical condition of the patient. Supplemental oxygen should be prescribed for those who have had thoracic or abdominal surgery, a history of ischaemic heart disease or respiratory insufficiency. The duration of oxygen therapy is determined on an individual basis so that a patient with angina having had gastric surgery should receive oxygen for at least 72 h after surgery. Any patient with a patient controlled analgesia (PCA) device should receive oxygen for the duration of use of the PCA.

- Analgesic regimens will be tailored to the type of surgery and physical status of the patient. Non-steroidal anti-inflammatory agents should be used with care in those with borderline renal function. If opioids are used then the dosing interval should be increased. Elderly patients can be safely given a PCA device on the ward, but should only receive one if they have the understanding and dexterity to use it. If the hospital has an acute pain team then patients with epidurals may be safely nursed on the general surgical ward. If no facility exists they should be cared for on a HDU as the elderly are more likely to get an inadvertent high block than younger patients.

- Age should not be a discriminator to admission to a HDU or ICU. Indeed if it is felt that major surgery will be of benefit to the patient then it seems perverse to deny them appropriate post-operative care. A recent debate in the literature was provoked by a case report[27] that documented the pre- and post-operative care of a 113 year old on an ICU. The majority of aged patients will be adequately cared for on a general surgical ward but a few will require post-operative HDU or ICU care which, providing that surgery was appropriate, should be readily available.

Further reading

Silverstein J. Geriatrics. *Anesthesiol Clin North Am* 2000; **18**: 1–209.

Jin F, Chung F. Minimizing perioperative adverse events in the elderly. *Br J Anaesth* 2001; **87**: 608–24.

McConachie I. Anaesthesia for the senior citizen. *Hospital Update* 1996; **22**: 82–91.

References

1. *The Office for National Statistics Population Trends.* Winter 2000, 2000. London: The Stationary Office.

2. Rodeheffer RJ, Gerstenblith G, Becker LC *et al.* Exercise cardiac output is maintained with advancing age in healthy human subjects: cardiac dilatation and increased stroke volume compensate for a diminished heart rate. *Circulation* 1984; **69 (2)**: 203–13.

3. Lakatta EG. Changes in cardiovascular function with aging. *Eur Heart J* 1990; **11 (suppl. C)**: 22–9.

4. Folkow B, Svanborg A. Physiology of cardiovascular aging. *Physiol Rev* 1993; **73**: 725–64.

5. Lakatta EG. Cardiovascular regulatory mechanisms in advanced age. *Physiol Rev* 1993; **73**: 413–67.

6. Priebe H-J. The aged cardiovascular risk patient. *Br J Anaesth* 2000; **85 (5)**: 763–78.

7. Peterson DD, Pack AI, Silage DA *et al.* Effects of aging on ventilatory and occlusion pressure responses to hypoxia and hypercapnia. *Am Rev Respir Dis* 1981; **124**: 387–91.

8. Wahba WM. Influence of aging on lung function – clinical significance of changes from age twenty. *Anesth Analg* 1983; **62**: 764–76.

9. Crapo RO, Campbell EJ. Aging of the respiratory system. In Fishman AP (ed.), *Pulmonary Diseases and Disorders.* New York, NY: McGraw-Hill, 1998; 251–64.

10. McLachlan MSF. The ageing kidney. *Lancet* 1978; **2**: 143–6.

11. Lindeman RD. Renal physiology and pathophysiology of aging. *Contrib Nephrol* 1993; **105**: 1–12.

12. Kampmann JP, Sinding J, Moller-Jorgensen I. Effect of age on liver function. *Geriatrics* 1975; **30**: 91–95.

13. Woodhouse KW, Mutch E, Williams FM *et al.* The effect of age on pathways of drug metabolism in human liver. *Age Ageing* 1984; **13**: 328–34.

14. Creasy H, Rapoport SI. The ageing human brain. *Ann Neurol* 1985; **17**: 2–10.

15. Dorfman LJ, Bosley TM. Age-related changes in peripheral and central nerve conduction in man. *Neurology* 1979; **29**: 38–44.

16. Collins KJ, Exton-Smith AN, James MH. Functional changes in autonomic nervous responses with ageing. *Age Ageing* 1980; **9**: 17–24.

17. Montamat SC, Cusack BJ, Vestal RE. Management of drug therapy in the elderly. *N Engl J Med* 1989; **231 (5)**: 303–9.

18. Variability in drug response. In Calvey TN, Williams NE (eds), *Principles and Practice of Pharmacology for Anaesthetists.* Oxford: Blackwell Scientific Publications, 1991; 133–5.

19. Extremes of age. *The 1999 report of the National Confidential Enquiry into Perioperative Deaths.* National CEPOD ISBN 0 95222069 6 X.

20. Then and now. *The 2000 report of the National Confidential Enquiry into Perioperative Deaths.* National CEPOD ISBN 0 9522069 7 8.

21. Kurz A, Plattner O, Sessler DI *et al.* The threshold for themoregulatory vaso-constriction during nitrous oxide/isoflurane anesthesia is lower in elderly than in young patients. *Anesthesiology* 1993; **79**: 465–9.

22. Frank SM, Shir Y, Raja SN *et al.* Core hypothermia and skin–surface temperature gradients. Epidural versus general anesthesia and the effects of age. *Anesthesiology* 1994; **80**: 502–8.

23. Rodgers A, Walker N, Schug S *et al.* Reduction in postoperative mortality and morbidity with epidural or spinal anaesthesia: results from overview of randomised trials. *Br Med J* 2000; **321**: 1493.

24. Knowles PR. Central nerve block and drugs affecting haemostasis – are they compatible? *Curr Anaesth Crit Care* 1996; **7**: 281–8.

25. Broadbent CR, Maxwell WB, Ferrie R *et al*. Ability of anaesthetists to identify a marked lumbar interspace. *Anaesthesia* 2000; **55 (11)**: 1122–6.

26. Greaves JD. Serious spinal cord injury due to haematomyelia caused by spinal anaesthesia in a patient treated with low-molecular weight heparin. *Anaesthesia* 1997; **52**: 150–4.

27. Oliver CD, White SA, Platt MW. Surgery for fractured femur and elective ICU admission at 113 yr of age. *Br J Anaesth* 2000; **84 (2)**: 260–2.

8

PERIOPERATIVE OPTIMISATION

Death rates from surgery and anaesthesia are now low. This is despite increasing complexity of the surgery performed and a rising average age of the population. However, just a small percentage of the patients undergoing surgery still carry most of the postoperative morbidity and mortality:

- Those most at risk are the elderly and those undergoing emergency surgery.

- Coexisting disease such as cardio-respiratory disease or diabetes mellitus further increases the chance of death.

The cause of death is most commonly from myocardial infarction or the gradual development of multiple organ failure syndrome (MODS), the median day of death being on the sixth postoperative day. The mechanisms of the development of MODS are still being elucidated. However, it is likely that it results from inflammatory cascades provoked by a multi-factorial aetiology that may include any combination of

- altered microcirculation causing tissue injury;

- ischaemia–reperfusion injury;

- direct surgical or traumatic tissue injury;

- surgical stimulation of metabolic and endocrine processes;

- blood loss and fluid shifts causing regional and global hypoperfusion;

- anaesthetic agents causing vasodilatation and altered regional blood flow;

- splanchnic hypoperfusion – this may be especially important since splanchnic blood may amount to two-fifths of the blood volume; damage to mucosal integrity and bacterial translocation may be important in initiating inflammatory cascades.

Many of these perioperative events have potential to cause an imbalance between oxygen delivery and demand, be it local or global. This is especially likely to occur in the presence of reduced physiological reserve where cardiac index (CI) cannot rise to meet the demand placed by surgery. The tissue hypoxia that results may precipitate the systemic inflammatory response syndrome (SIRS) that may then progress on to MODS.

If this is the case, then to reduce perioperative risk, we need to target those patients with limited physiological reserve and undergoing surgery of sufficient physiological insult.

IDENTIFYING PERIOPERATIVE RISK

In the scoring systems of Goldman and Detsky (see Chapter 1), particular risk is attached to poor cardiac reserve in the form of congestive cardiac failure, aortic stenosis and precarious myocardial perfusion.

This suggests the ability to meet the demands of surgery by maintaining or increasing perfusion and oxygen delivery might be important in determining survival:

- In support of this, early work by Boyd et al.[1] had suggested in cardiac surgery that failure to raise postoperative CI above $2.5 \, l/min/m^2$ was associated with increased mortality rate.

- Similarly, Clowes et al.[2] later showed that failure to increase cardiac output after thoracic surgery was associated with reduced survival.

- Shoemaker[3] also defined indicators of risk for perioperative death by correlating preoperative criteria with mortality rates (table 8.1). This work identified both patient criteria and criteria relating to the type of surgery to be undertaken. They and others subsequently used these criteria to identify and study high-risk patients.

Table 8.1 – Shoemaker's indicators of high risk.

Previous severe cardio-respiratory illness, e.g. acute myocardial infarction or chronic obstructive airways disease.
Extensive ablative surgery planned for malignancy, e.g. gastrectomy, oesophagectomy or surgery $> 6 \, h$.
Multiple trauma, e.g. more than three organ injuries, more than two systems or opening two body cavities.
Massive acute haemorrhage, e.g. > 8 units.
Age above 70 years and limited physiological reserve of one or more organs.
Septicaemia (positive blood cultures or septic focus) WCC > 13, pyrexia to 38.3 for 48 h.
Respiratory failure ($pO_2 < 8 \, kPa$ on an $FiO_2 > 0.4$ or mechanical ventilation $> 48 \, h$).
Acute abdominal catastrophe with haemodynamic instability (e.g. pancreatitis, perforated viscus, peritonitis, gastrointestinal bleed).
Acute renal failure (urea $> 20 \, mmol/l$, creatinine $> 260 \, mmol/l$).
Late stage vascular disease involving aortic disease.
Shock, e.g. MAP $< 60 \, mmHg$, CVP $< 15 \, cmH_2O$, urine output $< 20 \, ml/h$.

Improving outcome

Having identified the high-risk patient, how do we then set about improving outcome?

There are several potential strategies to consider:

- *Treatment of existing medical disease* – the principle of treating treatable medical conditions such as congestive cardiac failure, hypertension and respiratory disease is well established in anaesthetic practice, although the evidence for benefit, e.g. in moderate degrees of hypertension is limited.

- *Resuscitation of presenting disease* – where time allows attention should be directed to correcting electrolyte, metabolic and fluid balance. Circulating volume status and blood pressure should be restored using titrated fluid and inotropes.

- *Use of regional anaesthesia* – the use of regional anaesthesia has been shown to result in improved postoperative respiratory function. To date, however, there is little evidence to suggest that mortality rates are affected.

- *Strategies to prevent myocardial events* – beta blockers, nitrates, calcium channel blockers and alpha$_2$ antagonists have all been used to try to reduce postoperative mortality. In patients with ischaemic heart disease, there is some evidence of reductions in perioperative ischaemic events following administration of beta blockers.[4]

- *Cardio-respiratory optimisation* – there is increasing evidence to support the use of invasive monitoring, titrated fluids and inotropes to achieve enhanced cardiovascular function in anticipation of increased perioperative oxygen demand.

This evidence will be reviewed in the remainder of this chapter.

THE EVIDENCE FOR PERIOPERATIVE OPTIMISATION

The perioperative cardiovascular changes seen in high-risk patients undergoing major surgery were characterised in the 1970s by Shoemaker:

- In 1973, his group studied 98 patients undergoing major surgery and in variable levels of established shock. Comparing 67 survivors with 31 non-survivors, they were able to demonstrate significantly different haemodynamic changes in the days following surgery. Surviving patients had a higher CI, higher oxygen delivery and higher oxygen uptake. These indices were much better predictors of mortality than the more traditionally used values of blood pressure and heart rate.[5]

- Following this, the same group studied 220 high-risk patients this time undergoing major-elective and semi-elective surgery. In these patients, they confirmed higher values of CI, oxygen delivery and oxygen consumption in the survivors. From these findings, they postulated that if cardiovascular performance could be enhanced in high-risk patients to achieve the CI and oxygen delivery values manifest by survivors then overall survival rate could increase. They were able to suggest specific goals of CI ($4.5\,l/min/m^2$), oxygen delivery ($600\,ml/min/m^2$) and oxygen consumption ($170\,ml/min/m^2$) that they termed 'supranormal values'.[6]

- In a subsequent non-randomised study of 100 patients, they either actively increased cardiovascular performance with fluids and inotropes aiming to achieve the above supranormal values or in the control patients allowed CI to remain between 2.8 and $3.5\,l/min/m^2$. Mortality and complication rate were both reduced in the intervention group.[7]

Several other non-randomised studies confirmed these findings, however, it was not until the 1980s that further evidence was gained from properly randomised controlled trials:

- Firstly, in 1985 Schultz et al.[8] studied 70 patients undergoing surgical repair of hip fractures. Half of the patients were monitored with pulmonary artery flotation catheters and managed with intravenous fluids and inotropes to enhance CI and oxygen delivery to preset goals. The other half were managed conventionally. The intervention group had a significantly lower mortality rate by over 25%. It was unclear, however, whether the improvement was due to better monitoring or to enhanced oxygen delivery.

- Subsequently, in 1988 Shoemaker's group[9] published a randomised controlled trial of 340 high-risk surgical patients. They recruited patients using their previously defined criteria for high risk. Control patients were managed conventionally, whereas the protocol group were given intravenous fluids, inotropes and vasodilators aiming to achieve the supranormal values they had described previously. The protocol group had significantly lower mortality (4% vs 33% $p < 0.01$) and complication rate (1.3 vs 0.4 $p < 0.05$).

- Another group, Berlauk et al.,[10] published further data to support the use of perioperative optimisation. In this study, 89 patients underwent peripheral vascular surgery under general anaesthesia. Patients were randomised into three groups. One group received conventional management and the other two groups were monitored with a pulmonary artery catheter either placed 12 h before or immediately before surgery. In the latter two groups, the invasive monitoring was used to guide circulatory 'tune up' with fluid loading, inotropes and vasodilators. Treatment was given to maintain pulmonary capillary wedge pressure of 8–15 mmHg, CI $> 2.8\,l/min/m^2$ and SVR $< 1100\,dyne\,s/cm^5$ pre- and intraoperatively. The study groups both had fewer intraoperative adverse events, less early graft thrombosis and lower postoperative cardiac morbidity.

- In 1992 and 1995, Shoemaker's group published two further randomised controlled trials this time in 67 and 125 patients with severe trauma.[11,12] In patients treated to increase oxygen delivery to supranormal values, they found reduced organ failure, lower mortality rate, shorter stays in intensive care and shorter periods of ventilation.

- In a further randomised controlled trial, Boyd et al.[13] studied 107 patients at high risk as defined by Shoemaker's criteria. The majority of patients were admitted to intensive care preoperatively, although some were admitted postoperatively. All patients received conventional therapy with invasive monitoring, intravenous fluids, vasodilators and inotropes. The protocol group were managed in addition to deliberately increased oxygen delivery. Dopexamine was used to achieve goals of oxygen delivery of $> 600\,ml/min/m^2$ with pulmonary capillary wedge pressure 12–14 mmHg and haemoglobin $> 12\,g/l$. The result was a significantly lower mortality and complication rate (by 75% and 59%, respectively).

These impressive reductions in mortality and complication rates have not, however, been mirrored in some more recent randomised trials. Ziegler et al.[14] and Valentine et al.[15] both failed to show any significant benefit in terms of morbidity and mortality from optimisation attempts in patients undergoing peripheral vascular surgery.

Another recent study[16] of over 400 patients undergoing abdominal surgery using dopexamine also failed to show benefit.

It is possible that in at least some of these studies the targeted populations were not at high enough risk and therefore unlikely to show benefit from optimisation strategies. Clearly, the patients chosen for optimisation protocols need to be selected with care. Further, in one of these studies[15] the intraoperative complication rate was actually increased in the optimised group. Optimisation techniques should therefore be titrated with care to avoid inducing morbidity related to the therapy.

Another recent study by Wilson et al.[17] has added an exciting dimension to the concept of perioperative optimisation. In a randomised controlled trial of 138 patients they studied three high-risk groups undergoing surgery:

- The control group were managed conventionally and were admitted to intensive care if deemed necessary.

- The other two groups were admitted preoperatively to intensive care and given goal directed therapy with either adrenaline or dopexamine lasting for at least 12 h postoperatively.

- Both the treatment groups had significantly improved survival rate.

- However, only the dopexamine group saw a significant reduction in morbidity.

This is particularly interesting because the dopexamine treated group did not see an increase in CI by as much as the adrenaline treated group. The reduced morbidity was due to a reduction in sepsis and ARDS.

Dopexamine is a pure $beta_2$ agonist with very little $beta_1$ effect and no $alpha_1$ activity. Its inotropic effects result from inhibition of endogenous catecholamine reuptake and from stimulation of baroreceptor reflexes. It reduces systemic and pulmonary vascular resistance and increases both renal and splanchnic blood flow. $Beta_2$ stimulation also brings about anti-inflammatory properties. It may be that this together with improved splanchnic blood flow both maintains mucosal barriers and attenuates the inflammatory cascade that leads to SIRS and MODS. In support of this, dopexamine has been shown to reduce inflammatory change in the upper gastrointestinal mucosa in high-risk surgical patients.[18]

The specific benefits of dopexamine suggested in the study of Wilson *et al.* are by no means universally accepted. It has been suggested[19] that the three treatment groups in the study were not comparable and that this may have led to some of the differences seen between the dopexamine and adrenaline treated groups. Further work is therefore needed to establish the place of dopexamine.

The role of catecholamines and their actions at different adrenoceptors on the immune system is explored fully in a review cited in Further reading.

PATIENT SELECTION

There is accumulating evidence to suggest that the use of perioperative optimisation can improve postoperative outcome. The challenge is to identify

- those patients who will benefit,

- the appropriate goals to direct therapy to.

Table 8.1 lists Shoemaker's criteria for high-risk patients. However, we have seen that where perioperative risk is low there is little benefit from optimisation regimens. In fact, some studies have seen increased risk in optimised patients. In selecting patients who may benefit from optimisation, the anaesthetist must balance the risks of surgery and anaesthesia against possible detrimental effects of optimisation.

Shoemaker has also suggested therapeutic goals to target therapy to, the supranormal values described previously. Others have suggested that patients with initial oxygen delivery of $< 450\,ml/min/m^2$ should be targeted. Again it is probably a matter of judgement on the part of the anaesthetist to enhance cardiovascular function sufficiently to allow the demands of surgery to be met whilst at the same time not overstressing the myocardium and precipitating ischaemia or arrhythmia.

OPTIMISATION IN CRITICAL ILLNESS

Although there is good evidence to support the use of preoperative optimisation in elective and semi-elective surgery, there is unfortunately little to support the pursuit of supranormal goals for oxygen delivery in patients who are already critically ill:

- Initial non-randomised studies in patients with established septic shock[20] suggested that optimisation might be of benefit, however, subsequent randomised controlled trials have not supported this.

- A randomised study of patients with septic shock by Tuchshmidt et al.[21] found a reduced mortality rate in optimised patients but this was not significantly so.

- Other randomised studies[22–24] have all failed to show benefit from optimisation. All of these studies had in common the recruitment of patients with established septic shock and/or organ failure.

Another interesting study helps to clarify the situation:

- Gutierrez et al.[25] examined pHi as indicator of hypoperfusion at entry to their study. Those with a low pHi at entry to the study, suggesting existing hypoperfusion, did not benefit from optimisation whereas those without hypoperfusion at entry to the study did see reduced mortality.

It would appear that where organ failure is already established, there is little to gain from pursuing supranormal values.

Further reading

Uusaro A, Russell JA. Could anti-inflammatory actions of catecholamines explain the possible beneficial effects of supranormal oxygen delivery in critically ill surgical patients? *Inten Care Med* 2000; **26**: 299–304.

Kelly KM. Does increasing oxygen delivery improve outcome? Yes. *Crit Care Clin* 1996; **12**: 635–44.

Ronco JJ, Fenwick JC, Tweeddale MG. Does increasing oxygen delivery improve outcome in the critically ill? No. *Crit Care Clin* 1996; **12**: 645–59.

References

1. Boyd AR, Tremblay RE, Spencer FC *et al.* Estimation of cardiac output soon after intracardiac surgery with cardio–pulmonary bypass. *Ann Surg* 1959; **150**: 613.

2. Clowes GHA, Del Guercio LRM. Circulatory response to trauma of surgical operations. *Metabolism* 1960; **9**: 67.

3. Shoemaker WC, Czer LS. Evaluation of the biologic importance of various hemodynamic and oxygen transport variables: which variables should be monitored in postoperative shock? *Crit Care Med* 1979; **7**: 424.

4. Poldermans D, Boersma E, Bax JJ *et al.* The effect of bisoprolol on perioperative mortality and myocardial infarction in high-risk patients undergoing vascular surgery. Dutch Echocardiographic Cardiac Risk Evaluation Applying Stress Echocardiography Study Group. *N Engl J Med* 1999; **341**: 1789–94.

5. Shoemaker WC, Montgomery ES, Kaplan E *et al.* Physiologic patterns in surviving and nonsurviving shock patients. Use of sequential cardiorespiratory variables in defining criteria for therapeutic goals and early warning of death. *Arch Surg* 1973; **106**: 630.

6. Shoemaker WC, Pierchala C, Chang P *et al.* Prediction of outcome and severity of illness by analysis of the frequency distributions of cardiorespiratory variables. *Crit Care Med* 1977; **5**: 82.

7. Shoemaker WC, Appel PL, Waxman K *et al.* Clinical trial of survivors' cardiorespiratory patterns as therapeutic goals in critically ill postoperative patients. *Crit Care Med* 1982; **10**: 398.

8. Schultz RJ, Whitfield GF, LaMura *et al.* The role of physiologic monitoring in patients with fractures of the hip. *J Trauma* 1985; **25**: 309.

9. Shoemaker WC, Appel PL, Kram HB *et al.* Prospective trial of supranormal values of survivors as therapeutic goals in high-risk surgical patients. *Chest* 1988; **94**: 1176.

10. Berlauk JF, Abrams JH, Gilmour IJ *et al.* Preoperative optimization of cardiovascular hemodynamics improves outcome in peripheral vascular surgery. A prospective, randomized clinical trial. *Ann Surg* 1991; **214**: 289.

11. Fleming A, Bishop M, Shoemaker W *et al.* Prospective trial of supranormal values as goals of resuscitation in severe trauma. *Arch Surg* 1992; **127**: 1175.

12. Bishop MH, Shoemaker WC, Appel PL *et al.* Prospective, randomized trial of survivor values of cardiac index, oxygen delivery, and oxygen consumption as resuscitation endpoints in severe trauma. *J Trauma* 1995; **38**: 780.

13. Boyd O, Grounds RM, Bennett ED. A randomized clinical trial of the effect of deliberate perioperative increase of oxygen delivery on mortality in high-risk surgical patients. *JAMA* 1993; **270**: 2699.

14. Ziegler DW, Wright JG, Choban PS *et al.* A prospective randomized trial of preoperative 'optimization' of cardiac function in patients undergoing elective peripheral vascular surgery. *Surgery* 1997; **122**: 584.

15. Valentine RJ, Duke ML, Inman MH *et al.* Effectiveness of pulmonary artery catheters in aortic surgery: a randomized trial. *J Vasc Surg* 1998; **27**: 203.

16. Takala J, Meier-Hellmann A, Eddleston J *et al.* Effect of dopexamine on outcome after major abdominal surgery: a prospective, randomized, controlled multicenter study. European Multicenter Study Group on Dopexamine in Major Abdominal Surgery. *Crit Care Med* 2000; **28**: 3417.

17. Wilson J, Woods I, Fawcett J *et al.* Reducing the risk of major elective surgery: randomised controlled trial of preoperative optimisation of oxygen delivery. *Br Med J* 1999; **318**: 1099.

18. Byers RJ, Eddleston JM, Pearson RC *et al.* Dopexamine reduces the incidence of acute inflammation in the gut mucosa after abdominal surgery in high-risk patients. *Crit Care Med* 1999; **27**: 1787.

19. Snowden C, Roberts D. More than an abstract: 'To optimise or not to optimise that is the question'. *CPD Anaes* 2000; **2**: 43.

20. Edwards JD, Brown GC, Nightingale P *et al.* Use of survivors' cardiorespiratory values as therapeutic goals in septic shock. *Crit Care Med* 1989; **17**: 1098.

21. Tuchschmidt J, Fried J, Astiz M *et al.* Elevation of cardiac output and oxygen delivery improves outcome in septic shock. *Chest* 1992; **102**: 216.

22. Hayes MA, Yau EH, Timmins AC *et al.* Response of critically ill patients to treatment aimed at achieving supranormal oxygen delivery and consumption. Relationship to outcome. *Chest* 1993; **103**: 886.

23. Yu M, Levy MM, Smith P *et al.* Effect of maximizing oxygen delivery on morbidity and mortality rates in critically ill patients: a prospective, randomized, controlled study. *Crit Care Med* 1993; **21**: 830.

24. Gattinoni L, Brazzi L, Pelosi P *et al.* A trial of goal-oriented hemodynamic therapy in critically ill patients. SvO$_2$ Collaborative Group. *N Engl J Med* 1995; **333**: 1025.

25. Gutierrez G, Palizas F, Doglio G *et al.* Gastric intramucosal pH as a therapeutic index of tissue oxygenation in critically ill patients. *Lancet* 1992; **339**: 195.

9

THE PATIENT WITH CORONARY HEART DISEASE

Coronary heart disease (CHD) is widely prevalent in the adult population of the United Kingdom and is a major cause of morbidity and mortality:[1]

- In the surgical population, cardiovascular disease is the leading cause of death within 30 days of a surgical procedure, responsible for 36% of peri-operative deaths in the latest NCEPOD report.[2]

- Longer-term morbidity and mortality is also increased in patients with or at risk for CHD who undergo non-cardiac surgery.[3]

The management of the patient with CHD who requires anaesthesia for non-cardiac surgery is therefore an important issue for all anaesthetists.

PATHOPHYSIOLOGY

The major pathological feature in the patient with CHD is the presence of lipid atheromatous plaques within the walls of the epicardial coronary arteries. This feature, exacerbated sometimes by coronary arterial spasm, may lead to:

- Myocardial ischaemia when myocardial oxygen demand exceeds a limited myocardial oxygen supply; manifest clinically as stable angina.

- Rupture of plaque with thrombus formation leading to near or complete coronary arterial occlusion; manifest clinically as unstable angina, myocardial infarction or sudden cardiac death (the acute coronary syndromes).

In the patient who undergoes surgery, a number of profound stresses, including surgical trauma to tissue, marked changes in temperature, alteration of major organ function and the stress and inflammatory responses, combine to produce a range of pathophysiological derangements which, in the presence of CHD, may lead to myocardial injury in the peri-operative period.

- Sympathetic activity may result in myocardial oxygen supply/demand imbalance leading to myocardial ischaemia, and/or plaque instability and rupture.

- The inflammatory response may result in activation of vascular endothelium leading to plaque instability and rupture, and/or coronary arterial spasm.

- Changes in platelet function, and in the coagulation and fibrinolytic systems, predispose to coronary arterial thrombosis.

The patient with CHD who requires major surgery is thus at risk of myocardial injury which may become manifest in the immediate or delayed post-operative period as myocardial ischaemia or infarction, serious arrhythmias, ventricular failure or sudden cardiac death.

PRE-OPERATIVE MANAGEMENT

Aims

- Identification of the patient with severe CHD.

- Consideration of revascularisation and/or modification of medical therapy.

Identification of the patient with severe CHD

Guidelines for the pre-operative cardiac assessment of patients undergoing non-cardiac surgery have been published by the American College of Cardiology in conjunction with the American Heart Association.[4] A cardiological perspective on these matters is given in a later chapter:

- The identification of the patient with severe CHD is based upon an evaluation of information obtained from the history, examination and resting electrocardiogram.

- The identification of a patient with an acute coronary syndrome clearly mandates the postponement of elective or scheduled surgery and the immediate introduction of the appropriate medical therapy.

- In the majority of patients, however, the pre-operative assessment allows the identification of clinical markers associated with the presence of underlying severe CHD and with a high peri-operative and long-term cardiac risk.

The following clinical markers are most important:[5]

- symptoms of myocardial ischaemia (stable angina),

- history of previous myocardial infarction,

- congestive cardiac failure,

- diabetes mellitus.

In patients with several or all of these clinical markers, there is a high probability of severe CHD (left main stem disease, three vessel disease, or two vessel disease with involvement of the proximal left anterior descending artery), whilst in patients with none of these clinical markers, the risk of severe underlying CHD is less than 5%.[6] The effect of these clinical markers on peri-operative and long-term cardiac risk is similar – in patients undergoing vascular surgery who have none of these clinical markers, the combined incidence of peri-operative myocardial infarction and cardiac death is approximately 3%, whilst in patients with three or more of these markers, the risk is between 15% and 20%.[7]

The requirement for further cardiac investigation in a patient with the above clinical markers for CHD should be determined by a balanced assessment of the functional capacity of the patient and the cardiac risk (risk of myocardial infarction or cardiac death) associated with the specific surgical procedure to be performed.

The cardiac risk for non-cardiac surgical procedures has been stratified into high, intermediate and low risk groups:[4]

High cardiac risk ($>$ 5% mortality):

- major emergency surgery, particularly in the elderly,

- aortic and peripheral vascular surgery,

- anticipated prolonged procedures associated with large fluid shifts and/or blood loss.

Intermediate cardiac risk ($<$ 5% mortality):

- carotid endarterectomy,

- head and neck surgery,

- intraperitoneal and intrathoracic surgery,

- orthopaedic surgery,

- prostate surgery.

Low cardiac risk ($<$ 1% mortality):

- endoscopic procedures,

- superficial procedures,

- cataract surgery,

- breast surgery.

In general, in the presence of clinical markers for severe CHD, a patient who is to undergo high risk surgery requires further pre-operative cardiac investigation, whilst a patient who is to undergo low risk surgery does not require further pre-operative cardiac investigation.

Further pre-operative cardiac investigation is based on the identification of reversible myocardial ischaemia by one of a variety of methods of non–invasive testing:

- exercise stress electrocardiography,
- pharmacological stress electrocardiography,
- ambulatory electrocardiography,
- stress echocardiography,
- myocardial perfusion imaging.

In most ambulatory patients, the investigation of choice is exercise stress electro-cardiography, which can provide an estimate of functional capacity and detect myocardial ischaemia through changes in the electrocardiograph and the haemo-dynamic response. Pharmacological stress electrocardiography is appropriate in those patients unable to exercise for non–cardiac reasons, and stress echocardio-graphy or myocardial perfusion imaging appropriate in those patients with an abnormality of the resting electrocardiogram such as bundle branch block.

Invasive testing by coronary angiography is appropriate in the following groups of patients who are to undergo non–cardiac surgery:[8]

- patients with a high risk result during non–invasive testing,
- patients with myocardial ischaemia unresponsive to adequate medical therapy,
- patients with an acute coronary syndrome,
- patients with equivocal non–invasive testing who are to undergo high risk non–cardiac surgery.

The adoption of this structured approach will identify the majority of patients requiring non–cardiac surgery who have severe CHD. However, there remains no reasonable way to absolutely eliminate the possibility that an individual patient may suffer a cardiac complication during or after a surgical procedure.

Consideration of revascularisation and/or modification of medical therapy

Prophylactic coronary artery bypass grafting (CABG) prior to a non–cardiac elective surgical procedure is appropriate only in those patients who fulfil standard criteria for CABG surgery for prognostic reasons independent of the non-cardiac procedure:[9]

- suitable viable myocardium with left main stem disease,

- three vessel coronary artery disease with left ventricular dysfunction,

- two vessel coronary artery disease including left anterior descending disease with left ventricular dysfunction,

- myocardial ischaemia unresponsive to maximal medical therapy.

Although successful myocardial revascularisation by CABG surgery in other groups almost normalises non-cardiac peri-operative risk, this benefit is lost by the cumulative morbidity and mortality of the cardiac and the non-cardiac surgical procedures. The role of prophylactic percutaneous transluminal coronary angioplasty (PTCA) prior to a non-cardiac elective surgical procedure is less clearly defined as there is no evidence of prognostic benefit for angioplasty over medical therapy.[10] PTCA, in this setting, should be restricted to patients with reversible myocardial ischaemia in whom a single coronary arterial stenosis subtends a large area of viable myocardium:

- The majority of patients with CHD presenting for elective non-cardiac surgery do not have disease severe enough to justify the risks of coronary angiography and coronary revascularisation.

- In these patients, the optimisation of pre-operative medical therapy and the continuation of this medical regimen through the operative and post-operative periods is most appropriate.

Patients with CHD should be receiving one or more of the following medications for symptom control and/or prophylaxis, unless contraindicated:

- beta blockers,

- calcium channel blockers,

- nitrates,

- potassium channel activators,

- aspirin,

- angiotensin converting enzyme inhibitors or angiotensin receptor antagonists for patients with left ventricular dysfunction.

Beta blockers, calcium channel blockers, nitrates and the potassium channel activator nicorandil all limit the degree of myocardial ischaemia during exercise testing and may be expected to be of value peri-operatively.[11] Aspirin has a proven role in the primary and secondary prevention of myocardial infarction, mediated by its antiplatelet actions, and may be expected to be useful in the peri-operative period when platelet reactivity is increased.[12] Angiotensin converting enzyme inhibitors and angiotensin receptor antagonists reduce morbidity and mortality in patients with CHD and left ventricular dysfunction.[13]

The strongest evidence supports the peri-operative use of beta blockers, whose introduction should be considered in all patients with CHD, or risk factors for CHD, who require surgery:

- Beta blockers limit the chronotropic and inotropic effects of the increased sympathetic activity present in the peri-operative period, reducing myocardial oxygen requirements and increasing myocardial oxygen supply by increasing diastolic coronary perfusion time.

- They also limit the shear stress across atheromatous plaques in the coronary circulation and so may reduce the incidence of plaque rupture and consequent coronary arterial thrombosis.

- Beta blockers have been demonstrated to reduce the amount of myocardial ischaemia detected by ST segment analysis when administered peri-operatively.[14]

- Recent studies have indicated that the prophylactic use of beta blockers in the peri-operative period in patients with CHD, or risk factors for CHD, undergoing non-cardiac surgery reduces cardiac risk in the immediate and delayed post-operative periods.[15,16]

The direct evidence to support the introduction of calcium channel blockers, nitrates and the potassium channel activator nicorandil in the peri-operative period is less certain. Furthermore, these medications may produce vasodilatation and reflex tachycardia which may compromise myocardial perfusion in the patient with CHD undergoing anaesthesia and surgery. These agents should probably be reserved for patients who have previously required these medications for control of myocardial ischaemia, or for patients who develop myocardial ischaemia after surgery despite the appropriate use of a beta blocker.

The use of aspirin in the patient undergoing major surgery is limited by the perception that surgical bleeding is increased. However, aspirin has no effect on platelet aggregation induced by tissue collagen and should not, in theory, increase the risk of surgical bleeding.[17] The prophylactic use of aspirin should be considered, therefore, in the patient with CHD undergoing major surgery.

Angiotensin converting enzyme inhibitors and angiotensin receptor antagonists are vasodilators, which may interact with anaesthetic agents and techniques to produce profound hypotension and compromise myocardial perfusion. These medications are best avoided in the peri-operative period.

ANAESTHETIC CONSIDERATIONS IN THE PATIENT WITH SEVERE CHD

Aims

- Optimisation of pre-operative status by appropriate investigation, revascularisation and introduction of anti-ischaemic medical therapy.

- Preservation of the balance between myocardial oxygen supply and demand throughout the peri-operative period.

Optimisation of pre-operative status

The optimisation of pre-operative status and the need to continue the appropriate medical therapy throughout the peri-operative period has been discussed in the previous section. However, the degree of urgency of the non-cardiac surgical procedure may limit the amount of time that is available for pre-operative investigation and management. (NCEPOD classification of surgical urgency is discussed in Chapter 3):

- There is clearly no opportunity in the patient who requires emergency surgery for pre-operative investigation or therapy, and attention should be directed towards intensive cardiovascular monitoring and preservation of the myocardial oxygen supply and demand balance in the operative and post-operative periods, and to the introduction of appropriate anti-ischaemic medication in the post-operative period.

- Similarly, in the patient who requires urgent surgery, there is little time for the optimisation of pre-operative status.

- In the patient with an acute coronary syndrome who requires urgent non-cardiac surgery, consideration may be given to the use of an intra-aortic balloon pump device, in those centres which have cardiology or cardiac surgery support, in order to reduce myocardial oxygen requirements and to improve coronary perfusion and, thus, myocardial oxygen supply.[18]

- There is sufficient time in the patient requiring scheduled or elective surgery for the appropriate optimisation of pre-operative status.

- It may become necessary to delay scheduled surgery if the patient is found to have CHD necessitating revascularisation according to the criteria discussed previously.

- Occasionally, the use of an intra-aortic balloon pump may be considered in those patients demonstrated to have severe CHD not amenable to revascularisation.

- Current recommendations indicate that a patient who has suffered an uncomplicated myocardial infarction may undergo scheduled non-cardiac surgery four weeks after the myocardial infarction providing rigorous haemodynamic monitoring and control is applied throughout the peri-operative period.[4,19]

However, persisting myocardial ischaemia after infarction, which should be sought by non-invasive testing, is an indication for invasive investigation which will delay surgery further if revascularisation should be proved necessary.

- The patient who has suffered an uncomplicated myocardial infarction who requires elective non-cardiac surgery should wait for at least 3 months before undergoing surgery in order to minimise the risk of peri-operative myocardial infarction.[20]

Preservation of myocardial oxygen supply and demand

The essence of anaesthetic management in the patient with severe CHD under-going non-cardiac surgery is the preservation of the balance between myocardial oxygen supply and demand.

Myocardial oxygen supply is determined by

- coronary artery blood flow,
- arterial oxygen content.

Coronary artery blood flow is dependent on

- coronary perfusion pressure (CPP), determined by the aortic diastolic pressure minus the left ventricular end diastolic pressure (LVEDP);
- coronary vascular resistance, determined by blood viscosity, sympathetic tone and, most importantly in the patient with CHD, fixed resistance due to coronary atheromatous disease;
- duration of diastole determined by the heart rate (shorter diastole with faster heart rates).

Coronary artery blood flow is directly related to the CPP, and inversely related to the coronary vascular resistance and the heart rate.

Arterial oxygen content is dependent on

- haemoglobin concentration,
- haemoglobin saturation,
- arterial oxygen tension.

Myocardial oxygen demand is determined by

- heart rate,

- left ventricular afterload,

- left ventricular preload,

- myocardial contractility.

In the patient with severe CHD, the myocardial oxygen demand must not be allowed to outstrip the supply.

Increased myocardial oxygen demand	Decreased myocardial oxygen supply
Tachycardia	Tachycardia
Increased afterload	Decreased aortic diastolic pressure
Increased preload (LVEDP)	Increased LVEDP
Increased contractility	Decreased arterial oxygen content

- Tachycardia and an increased LVEDP have greater potential to induce myocardial ischaemia as both increase demand and reduce supply, than hypertension which increases demand, but also supply due to the associated increase in aortic diastolic pressure resulting in an increased CPP.

- Hypotension, with a decreased aortic diastolic pressure, in association with tachycardia and/or increased LVEDP is a particularly hazardous combination of haemodynamic change that must be avoided in the patient with severe CHD.

Monitoring

An essential prerequisite for the preservation of the balance between myocardial oxygen supply and demand is the establishment of a level of monitoring appropriate to the disease severity of the patient and the magnitude of the surgery. The Association of Anaesthetists of Great Britain and Ireland has stated that the following patient monitoring devices are essential to the safe conduct of anaesthesia for all patients:[21]

- electrocardiograph,

- non-invasive arterial pressure monitoring,

- pulse oximetry,

- capnography,

- vapour analysis.

This level of monitoring is sufficient in the majority of patients with severe CHD undergoing low risk surgery but must be supplemented by additional monitoring for patients undergoing intermediate or high risk surgery:

- invasive cardiovascular monitoring,
- temperature,
- urine output.

Invasive cardiovascular monitoring includes arterial and central venous pressure monitoring. The use of pulmonary artery catheterisation is controversial but is likely to be of benefit in the following groups of patients:[22]

- patients with a recent myocardial infarction,
- patients with significant CHD undergoing high risk surgical procedures,
- patients with CHD and associated left ventricular dysfunction undergoing intermediate risk surgical procedures.

Anaesthetic techniques

There is no evidence to demonstrate a consistent advantage of any general anaesthetic agent or technique over any other, in relation to the risk of peri-operative cardiac morbidity and mortality. Several large studies of patients undergoing CABG have demonstrated no difference in outcome with differing anaesthetic agents e.g. volatile agents versus narcotic based techniques.

All anaesthetic agents and techniques are associated with cardiovascular effects, and the care with which the chosen agent and/or technique is managed is more important than the choice of agent or technique itself. Particular attention should, however, be directed to control of the haemodynamic changes associated with the following interventions:

- induction of anaesthesia,
- laryngoscopy and tracheal intubation,
- surgical incision and stimulation,
- emergence from anaesthesia,
- tracheal extubation.

Many pharmacological approaches are available to obtund the haemodynamic response to airway manipulation, including the use of opioids or cardiovascular medications such as beta blockers.[23] Alternatively, the haemodynamic response to airway manipulation can be minimised by the use of a laryngeal mask airway rather than an endotracheal tube, when this is otherwise appropriate.

Regional anaesthesia may be used as an adjunct or as an alternative to general anaesthesia. However, the available evidence in high risk patients undergoing lower extremity vascular surgery indicates that carefully conducted epidural anaesthesia and general anaesthesia are associated with comparable rates of cardiac morbidity.[24] If a regional anaesthetic technique is to be employed, it is essential that attention is directed to the avoidance of sudden and severe hypotension and the potential decrease in coronary perfusion associated with the technique, and consequently, epidural catheter techniques are to be preferred to subarachnoid single-shot techniques.

Detection of intra-operative myocardial ischaemia

Methods of peri-operative surveillance for myocardial ischaemia include:

- computerised ST segment monitoring,
- pulmonary artery pressure monitoring,
- transoesophageal echocardiography.

Computerised ST segment trend analysis is superior to visual interpretation of ST segment changes for the detection of intra-operative and post-operative myocardial ischaemia and should be used if available. Similarly, changes in pulmonary artery pressure and pulmonary artery occlusion pressure and waveform can be sensitive indicators of myocardial ischaemia. Transoesophageal echocardiography, by the detection of wall motion abnormalities, is a further method in appropriately trained hands for the detection of intra-operative myocardial ischaemia.

Management of intraoperative ischaemia

Management of intra-operative myocardial ischaemia should concentrate on:

- The correction of haemodynamic status by manipulation of the depth of anaesthesia and the use of vasoactive agents. Beta blockers may be used to slow the heart rate and, thereby, to limit myocardial oxygen demand and increase myocardial oxygen supply. The rapid onset and titratability of the intravenous beta blocker esmolol make this a particularly suitable agent for use in this role.

- The use of intravenous nitroglycerin which appears to redistribute myocardial blood flow and may reverse myocardial ischaemia.

POST-OPERATIVE CARE

- The importance of continuing these principles of care into the post-operative period is increasingly apparent.

- Numerous studies indicate that with modern anaesthetic techniques, the occurence of intra-operative myocardial ischaemia can be limited, but that post-operative myocardial ischaemia remains common and is associated with the development of significant cardiac morbidity and mortality.[25]

Post-operative care should concentrate on the maintenance of

- adequate oxygenation,

- normothermia,

- haemodynamic stability requiring the continuation of invasive cardio-vascular monitoring,

- fluid balance,

- appropriate pain control based upon regional anaesthetic or systemic opioid analgesic techniques,

- administration of anti-ischaemic medical therapy.

The appropriate location for such care is an intensive care or high dependency care environment.

Further reading

Ramsay J. The patient with heart disease. *Can J Anaesth* 1996; **43**: R99–107.

Foex, Howell SJ. The myocardium. *Can J Anaesth* 1997; **44**: R67–76.

Nugent M. Anesthesia and myocardial ischemia. *Anesth Analg* 1992; **75**: 1–3.

References

1. Department of Health. *The National Service Framework for Coronary Heart Disease.* Stationery Office, London, 2000.

2. Callum KG, Gray AJG, Hoile RW *et al.* Then and now. *The 2000 report of the National Confidential Enquiry into Perioperative Deaths.* Royal College of Surgeons, London, 2000.

3. Mangano DT, Browner WS, Hollenberg M, Tateo IM. Long term cardiac prognosis following non-cardiac surgery. The study of Perioperative Ischemia Research Group. *JAMA* 1992; **268**: 233–9.

4. Guidelines for perioperative cardiovascular evaluation for noncardiac surgery. Report of the American College of Cardiology/American Heart Association Task Force on practice guidelines (Committee on Perioperative Cardiovascular Evaluation for Noncardiac Surgery). *JACC* 1996; **27**: 910–48.

5. Eagle KA, Coley CM, Newell JB *et al.* Combining clinical and thallium data optimizes preoperative assessment of cardiac risk before major vascular surgery. *Ann Intern Med* 1989; **110**: 859–66.

6. Paul SD, Eagle KA, Kuntz KM *et al.* Concordance of preoperative clinical risk with angiographic severity of coronary artery disease in patients undergoing vascular surgery. *Circulation* 1996; **94**: 1561–6.

7. L'Italien GJ, Paul SD, Hendel RC *et al.* Development and validation of a Bayesian model for perioperative cardiac risk assessment in a cohort of 1,081 vascular surgical candidates. *JACC* 1996; **27**: 779–86.

8. Guidelines for coronary angiography. Report of the American College of Cardiology/American Heart Association Task Force on assessment of diagnostic and therapeutic cardiovascular procedures (Subcommittee on Coronary Angiography). *JACC* 1987; **10**: 935–50.

9. Guidelines and indications for coronary artery bypass graft surgery. Report of the American College of Cardiology/American Heart Association Task Force on assessment of diagnostic and therapeutic cardiovascular procedures (Subcommittee on Coronary Artery Bypass Graft Surgery). *JACC* 1991; **17**: 543–89.

10. Guidelines for percutaneous transluminal coronary angioplasty. Report of the American College of Cardiology/American Heart Association Task Force on assessment of diagnostic and therapeutic cardiovascular procedures (Subcommittee on Percutaneous Transluminal Coronary Angioplasty). *JACC* 1993; **22**: 2033–54.

11. Jackson G. Stable angina: drugs, angioplasty or surgery? *Eur Heart J* 1997; **18**: B2–10.

12. Antiplatelet Trialists' Collaboration. Collaborative overview of randomised trials of antiplatelet therapy-1: prevention of death, myocardial infarction, and stroke by prolonged antiplatelet therapy in various categories of patients. *Br Med J* 1994; **308**: 81–106.

13. Pfeffer MA, Braunwald E, Ciampi A *et al.* Effect of captopril on mortality and morbidity in patients with left ventricular dysfunction after myocardial infarction. Results of the survival and enlargement trial. *N Engl J Med* 1992; **327**. 669–77.

14. Pasternack PF, Grossi EA, Baumann FG *et al.* Beta blockade to decrease silent myocardial ischaemia during peripheral vascular surgery. *Am J Surg* 1989; **158**: 113–16.

15. Mangano DT, Layug EL, Wallace A, Tateo IM. Effect of atenolol on mortality and cardiovascular morbidity after noncardiac surgery. *N Engl J Med* 1996; **335**: 1713–20.

16. Poldermans D, Boersma E, Bax JJ *et al*. The effect of bisoprolol on perioperative mortality and myocardial infarction in high-risk patients undergoing vascular surgery. *N Engl J Med* 1999; **341**: 1789–94.

17. Packham MA. Role of platelets in thrombosis and haemostasis. *Can J Physiol Pharmacol* 1994; **72**: 575–80.

18. Siu SC, Kowalchuk GJ, Welty FK *et al*. Intra-aortic balloon counterpulsation support in the high risk patient undergoing urgent noncardiac surgery. *Chest* 1991; **99**: 1342–5.

19. Shah KB, Kleinman BS, Sami H *et al*. Reevaluation of perioperative myocardial infarction in patients with prior myocardial infarction undergoing noncardiac operations. *Anesth Analg* 1990; **71**: 231–5.

20. Goldman L. Cardiac risk in noncardiac surgery: an update. *Anesth Analg* 1995; **80**: 810–20.

21. Association of Anaesthetists of Great Britain and Ireland. *Recommendations for Standards of Monitoring during Anaesthesia and Recovery*, 2000.

22. Practice guidelines for pulmonary artery catheterization. A report by the American Society of Anesthesiologists Task Force on pulmonary artery catheterization. *Anesthesiology* 1993; **78**: 229–30.

23. Ng WS. Pathophysiological effects of tracheal intubation. In Latto IP, Vaughan RS (eds), *Difficulties in Tracheal Intubation*. London: WB Saunders, 1997.

24. Christopherson R, Beattie C, Frank SM *et al*. Perioperative morbidity in patients randomized to epidural or general anesthesia for lower extremity vascular surgery. Perioperative Ischemia Randomized Anesthesia Trial Study Group. *Anesthesiology* 1993; **79**: 422–34.

25. Mangano DT, Browner WS, Hollenberg M *et al*. Associations of perioperative myocardial ischemia with cardiac morbidity and mortality in men undergoing noncardiac surgery. *N Engl J Med* 1990; **323**: 1781–8.

10

VALVULAR HEART DISEASE AND PULMONARY HYPERTENSION

This chapter aims to provide an outline of the management of patients with valvular heart disease with or without pulmonary hypertension, who are undergoing non-cardiac surgery:

- Not much data exists regarding valvular heart disease and perioperative risk analysis.

- The presence of ventricular dysfunction, arrhythmia, pulmonary hypertension, and coexisting coronary artery disease all contribute to cardiac risk.

- Published data is conflicting; however, there is consensus that aortic stenosis (AS) is a strong independent predictor of perioperative risk. Aortic incompetence (AI) has also been associated with increased perioperative mortality. The risks of mitral stenosis (MS) and mitral regurgitation (MR) are less clear. It would appear that in the absence of heart failure or recent myocardial infarction, lesions of the mitral valve do not contribute significantly to perioperative mortality. It is, however, very important to note that all of these four valve lesions *are* associated with an increased incidence of postoperative congestive heart failure.

In order to minimise risk to patients, all anaesthetists should undertake as meticulous a preoperative assessment as possible and plan the anaesthetic according to individual patient's diseases and the urgency and nature of the planned surgery. Anaesthetic planning should include appropriate investigations, premedication and plans for the conduct of anaesthesia, including monitoring techniques, analgesic strategies and plans for the postoperative management of these patients.

Awareness of the pathophysiological processes involved in valvular heart disease and pulmonary hypertension is essential to the successful anaesthetic management of patients presenting for non-cardiac surgery. Anticipation of the effects of surgical stresses including blood loss and other interventions such as the introduction of pneumoperitoneum during laparoscopy, alterations in position, application of tourniquets to limbs or cross-clamps to large blood vessels and the reperfusion associated with their release will surely facilitate in reducing morbidity and mortality in these high-risk surgical patients.

MONITORING

It is essential that appropriate monitoring be instituted before the induction of any form of anaesthesia in these high-risk patients. In addition to routine standard monitoring, anaesthetists should have a very low threshold for using direct arterial blood pressure monitoring. Central venous pressure (CVP) monitoring and the use of a pulmonary artery flotation catheter (PAFC), in particular, may assist in monitoring fluid therapy. It must be borne in mind, however, that arrhythmias can be induced by the insertion of guide wires and catheters into the heart. Ventricular arrhythmias, in particular, are sometimes difficult to treat in patients with severe ventricular hypertrophy, and a defibrillator should be present whenever such procedures are being undertaken. Where the expertise is available, trans-oesophageal echocardiography (TOE) can be a very useful adjunct to monitoring, and can be used to guide volume replacement, as well as to monitor ventricular performance. Institutional facilities and expertise will inevitably vary, and monitoring should be appropriate to the ability to interpret the information obtained.

AORTIC STENOSIS

Definitions

The severity of AS is traditionally estimated at cardiac catheterisation, and expressed as the peak-to-peak pressure gradient (PG) between the left ventricle (LV) and the aorta, PG = P (LV) − P (aorta):

- A PG greater than 50 mmHg is defined as critical AS.

It is important to remember that this value is true for patients with normal cardiac output, and smaller gradients may occur in those who have LV failure, and worse degrees of AS. It is possible to quantify PGs using Doppler echocardiography, however, patients older than 50 should have coronary angiography to exclude concomitant coronary artery disease.

Valve surface area (the area of the orifice of the open valve) is also an important measurement in AS. The normal valve surface area is 2.6–3.5 cm^2. A valve surface area of 1 cm^2 or less is likely to cause clinically significant aortic valve obstruction.

Aetiology and risk

Isolated AS is usually an acquired disease. Degeneration and/or calcification may occur on a previously normal valve, or on a congenitally bicuspid valve. The end result is obstruction of the aortic outflow. Isolated rheumatic disease of the aortic valve is not common:

- Presenting symptoms include angina, syncope, and heart failure.

- Onset of symptoms from AS is usually followed by death within 2–5 years if the diseased valve is not replaced.

Goldman found AS to be one of nine independent predictive variables that increased risk of perioperative cardiovascular morbidity.[1] However, O'Keefe has suggested that 'aggressive intraoperative monitoring and prompt recognition of haemodynamic abnormalities' can allow for safe anaesthesia in patients with severe, symptomatic AS undergoing non-cardiac surgery.[2] Selected patients with severe AS can therefore undergo non-cardiac surgery, but they are at greater risk, and demand appropriate monitoring and meticulous haemodynamic management during the perioperative time. Decisions to proceed with anaesthesia and surgery in these patients need to be made with due consideration of severity of AS, and relative urgency of proposed surgery. Certainly, patients with New York Heart Association (NYHA) class 4 symptoms, i.e. breathless at rest ought to have valvular surgery before elective non-cardiac surgery. Patients needing urgent or emergency surgery *may* benefit from valvuloplasty.

Pathophysiology

Obstructing the outflow of blood from the LV causes an increase in LV wall tension, with compensatory and characteristic concentric hypertrophy of the LV. This LV *pressure overload* induced hypertrophy results in reduced ventricular compliance, and higher end diastolic pressures are needed to fill the stiff LV. Patients with AS are particularly dependent on the contribution of atrial contraction to ventricular filling, hence atrial arrhythmias can produce critical loss of cardiac output and should be avoided at all costs.

End stage AS is associated with severe loss of compliance and the inability of the LV to sustain cardiac output, with loss of stroke volume as well as a reduced ejection fraction. This leads to a state known as *afterload mismatch*, with the heart failing because of excessive afterload, rather than contractility failure. Surgical correction of the high afterload by valve replacement replacing the valve should restore ejection fraction.

The hypertrophied myocardium in AS is vulnerable to ischaemia, because of increased oxygen demand and high wall tension. Even with normal coronary arteries, subendocardial ischaemia can occur, as coronary blood flow cannot keep pace with the ventricular hypertrophy. Tachycardia should be avoided as it aggravates ischaemia.

Pharmacological afterload reduction does not alleviate the mechanical afterload to the LV, and should be avoided as the associated reduction in diastolic blood pressure may cause myocardial ischaemia.

Conduct of anaesthesia

It may be reasonable to consider regional anaesthetic techniques, including epidural[3–5] and even continuous spinal[6] anaesthesia for selected patients with AS. However, the fall in diastolic blood pressure, and the potential bradycardia that may occur make these anaesthetic techniques potentially hazardous.

The choice of anaesthetic agents should be aimed at avoiding myocardial depression, and avoiding peripheral arteriolar vasodilation.

Certain haemodynamic objectives need to be met or maintained:

- The patient with AS should be kept well filled, with high normal filling pressures.

- The afterload should be maintained with judicious use of vasopressors.

- Tachycardia should be avoided.

- In particular, diastolic hypotension should be avoided, and falls in blood pressure should be corrected with volume replacement and alpha agonist drugs.

- Arrhythmias should be treated promptly by cardioversion in the event of haemodynamic compromise.

Appropriate observation and monitoring should be continued into the postoperative period.

Vasodilating and myocardial depressant induction agents (propofol and thiopentone) should best be avoided or used with great caution. Opiates are generally well tolerated, and may allow for reduced concentrations of inhalational anaesthetic agents. Vecuronium, cisatracurium, and rocuronium are all suitable muscle relaxants.

AORTIC INCOMPETENCE

Definitions

Incompetence of the aortic valve results in regurgitation of a portion of the stroke volume back into the LV during diastole. The severity of AI is quantified by the volume of regurgitant blood as estimated during angiography, or by colour flow

Doppler echocardiography. It may be mild, moderate or severe:

- Less than 3 l/min is deemed mild, and more than 6 l/min is severe AI.

- It is possible to have regurgitant volumes in excess of 20 l/min.

Aetiology

Disease of the valve leaflets, or the wall of the aortic root, or both can cause AI. Causes include: rheumatic fever, infective endocarditis, trauma, a congenitally bicuspid valve, failure of a bioprosthetic valve, and myxomatous disease of the aortic valve. AI can occur in the presence of ventricular septal defect, and as a consequence of aortic dissection. More rare causes include connective tissue diseases and congenital defects as well as treatment with the appetite suppressant phentermine–fenfluramine.

Pathophysiology

The regurgitant volume in chronic AI causes increased diastolic volume in the LV, which in turn provides a degree of haemodynamic compensation for the loss of forward stroke volume by the process of *preload augmentation*. Progression of the disease results in increased wall tension and *eccentric hypertrophy* of the LV. The heart can be grossly enlarged. The competent mitral valve protects the left atrium (LA) and pulmonary vasculature from the volume overload of AI. In severe AI, the regurgitant jet impinges on the anterior leaflet of the mitral valve and produces the presystolic mitral murmur of Austin Flint. The LV is initially very compliant, and unlikely to become ischaemic until late in the disease process when LV failure occurs. LV failure occurs when the chronically increased wall tension and muscle mass result in loss of compliance and contractility. The onset of LV failure is followed by rapid deterioration. Reduced afterload and moderate tachycardia are the chief mechanisms to offset the effects of AI.

A reduction in afterload as achieved by the lower diastolic aortic pressure augments forward flow. A faster heart rate (>90 beats/min) reduces diastolic time and hence the regurgitant fraction.

Acute AI is poorly tolerated and patients rapidly develop heart failure with distension of the LV and increased LA and pulmonary artery occlusion pressure (PAOP), as the mitral valve is unable to contain the regurgitant volume.

Conduct of anaesthesia

To minimise the effects of an incompetent aortic valve, the anaesthetic should aim to reduce or maintain a low afterload, and to keep a heart rate of about 90 beats/min. Regional anaesthesia is a logical choice where patients do not have any other contra-indications to its use. Bradycardia should be treated aggressively and in low cardiac output states dobutamine or milrinone are both reasonable choices if inotropic drugs are needed. Moderate vasodilation from both induction and inhalational anaesthetic agents may be beneficial to patients with AI.

MITRAL STENOSIS

Definitions

The normal mitral valve orifice in adults is between 4 and $6\,cm^2$:

- Clinically significant MS occurs when the valve orifice is less than $2\,cm^2$.

- When the mitral valve opening is reduced to $1\,cm^2$, the MS is said to be critical.

The diastolic trans–mitral PG can be accurately estimated by Doppler echocardiography. A gradient of

- less than $5\,mmHg$ is consistent with mild MS,

- 5–$12\,mmHg$ is consistent with moderate MS,

- greater than $12\,mmHg$ is severe MS.

Aetiology

Rheumatic heart disease is the most common cause of MS. Women are four times more likely to be affected than men. Congenital MS is rarely seen in infants and children. Malignant carcinoid, amyloid deposits, systemic lupus erythematosus, rheumatoid arthritis, and the Hunter Hurler mucopolysaccharidososes are other rare causes. Large vegetations from infective endocarditis of the mitral valve, as well as LA tumours (usually myxomas) and congenital membranes in the LA (cor triatriatum) may all mimic MS.

Pathophysiology

MS causes chronic under-filling of the LV, and results in increased pressure and volume upstream of the mitral valve. In order to generate adequate flow through a valve with a $1\,cm^2$ orifice to maintain a normal cardiac output, the LA pressure has to be approximately $25\,mmHg$. This increased LA pressure causes dilation of the LA and with disease progression, the pulmonary venous and capillary pressure increases. The pressure in the pulmonary arteries (PAs) also increases and medial hypertrophy occurs in these vessels. The right ventricle (RV) has to work harder and RV hypertrophy occurs. RV dysfunction and failure is a poor prognostic sign and secondary dysfunction of the right-sided valves (tricuspid and pulmonic regurgitation) occurs in severe MS.

For a given orifice size, the transvalvular PG is proportional to the square of the transvalvular flow rate. Therefore a doubling of flow rate will quadruple the PG.

Exercise, pregnancy, hypervolaemia, and hyperthyroidism or any other cause of increased cardiac output will significantly increase the transvalvular PG.

Atrial contraction contributes approximately 30% of ventricular filling in patients with MS. Atrial fibrillation (a common feature in MS with LA enlargement), therefore significantly decreases cardiac output. Tachycardia reduces diastolic time more than systolic time, thereby reducing the time available for flow across the mitral valve. This increases the transvalvular gradient and LA pressures further. Thus, atrial fibrillation should be aggressively managed and when it does occur, it is very important to control ventricular rate.

Conduct of anaesthesia

- The single most important aspect of the anaesthetic plan in patients with MS is to avoid tachycardia.

- Atrial fibrillation or tachycardia should be treated promptly by cardioversion or β blockade.

Filling pressures should be kept fairly high, but pulmonary oedma should be avoided. PA pressure monitoring may be desirable, as it can help to maintain optimal LA pressure, however, there is increased risk of PA rupture during balloon inflation, and the wedge pressure trace may not be attainable.

Afterload reduction should be avoided, as hypotension ensues with the stenotic mitral valve precluding compensatory increase in cardiac output to maintain blood pressure. LV function is usually normal, though it will be relatively small and non-compliant.

As with AS, it is advisable to avoid vasodilating induction agents and volatile agents should be used with caution and titrated carefully.

MITRAL REGURGITATION

Definitions

MR may be acute or chronic. Acute MR is usually a result of infection (endocarditis) or ischaemia with papillary muscle or chordal dysfunction. This usually requires urgent cardiac surgical intervention, and anaesthesia for these patients is beyond the scope of this chapter. Chronic MR is described as mild, moderate or severe. The quantification of MR is made by cine-angiography, and/or colour flow Doppler and pulsed wave Doppler echocardiography.

The volume of MR can be estimated from the difference between LV stroke volumes, measured during angiography, and the effective forward stroke volumes measured indirectly using the Fick method:

- In severe MR, the regurgitant stroke volume approaches or even exceeds forward stroke volume.

Echocardiographic quantification of severity of MR is made using Doppler colour flow mapping to estimate the size and volume of the regurgitant jet, and pulsed wave Doppler to observe flow reversal in the pulmonary veins as occurs in severe MR.

Echocardiography also provides useful information regarding the cause of MR and the dimensions of the LA.

Aetiology

Abnormalities of any of the components of the mitral valve apparatus can cause MR. This includes the mitral valve leaflets, the chordae tendineae, the papillary muscles, and the mitral annulus. Mitral leaflet pathology is usually of rheumatic origin, although endocarditis is also implicated. The mitral valve prolapse syndrome is another important cause. Rarely blunt or penetrating trauma may cause destruction of the mitral leaflets.

Chordal dysfunction may follow acute myocardial infarction or endocarditis. Ischaemia or infarction commonly causes posterior papillary muscle dysfunction.

Degenerative disease of the mitral annulus is common and is an important cause of MR particularly in female patients. Dilation of the annulus occurs in any cardiac disease associated with LV dilatation. It is particularly associated with ischaemic cardiomyopathy.

Pathophysiology

The pathophysiology of MR is best thought of in terms of chronic LV overload. The incompetent valve allows a proportion of the LV stroke volume back into the LA. The LA is highly compliant and may dilate to massive proportions. A significant proportion of the stroke volume will flow retrograde through the mitral valve before the aortic valve opens. The LV ejection fraction should therefore be increased (>80%). A normal ejection fraction (50–60%) may indicate depressed myocardial contractility. With large regurgitant volumes in the LA, pulmonary venous congestion ensues, and pulmonary arterial hypertension is a feature of chronic volume overload. The regurgitant fraction is influenced by LV afterload, the size of the regurgitant defect, the PG between the LA and LV as well as the heart rate. Moderate tachycardia reduces systole and the time for regurgitant blood flow, as well as reducing diastole and the time for diastolic filling of the LV. The absence of a competent mitral valve means that there is no isovolemic contraction phase during systole.

Conduct of anaesthesia

Anaesthetic goals include:

- avoid increases in afterload,
- maintain a relative tachycardia (about 90 beats/min),
- maintain relatively high filling pressures.

As with MS, excessive filling is bad and hypotension is best treated with inotropes rather than with vasopressors. PA catheters provide useful information, both in terms of pulmonary hypertension and the severity of MR, which may be seen as a 'v' wave on the PA wedge trace. Where inotropes are needed, both milrinone and dobutamine are logical choices as the reduction in afterload is augmented by the reduction in PA pressure. In the event of excessive loss of systemic vascular tone, judicious vasopressor (norepinephrine) infusion is appropriate to allow continued use of inotropes. Regional anaesthetic techniques are desirable, as the reduction in afterload, and the avoidance of the sympathetic surges associated with laryngoscopy are beneficial to the patient. Regional anaesthetic techniques should never excuse inadequate monitoring and vigilance.

PULMONARY HYPERTENSION

Definitions

Pulmonary hypertension is defined as PA systolic pressure greater than 30 mmHg and mean pressure greater than 20 mmHg. Pulmonary hypertension may be primary (idiopathic) or secondary.

Aetiology

Primary pulmonary hypertension is a rare but progressive and fatal disease. Secondary causes of pulmonary hypertension include MR, MS, LV diseases, pericardial diseases, LA myxomas, congenital cardiac defects, pulmonary embolism or thrombosis, pulmonary parenchymal disease, and chronic hypoxaemic states as well as some collagen vascular diseases.

Pathophysiology

Chronic resistance to pulmonary blood flow may cause secondary pulmonary hypertension. Otherwise, a reactive process may cause it. Increased resistance to flow often results in an additive reactive component. The effects of pulmonary hypertension and increased resistance to flow on the RV are complex. The RV is a thin walled structure whose function is highly influenced by its geometry. Chronically elevated PA pressures cause RV hypertrophy, which in turn results in loss of compliance and poor performance. RV failure is notoriously difficult to manage. Apart from the deleterious effects on RV function, the hydrostatic effects of pulmonary hypertension predispose to the development of pulmonary oedema and hypoxaemia from ventilation perfusion mismatch. The loss of RV compliance means that filling pressure in the RV is difficult to optimise – under filling leads to underperformance while the over-filled ventricle rapidly fails. Excessive distension of the RV also results in leftward displacement of the interventricular septum, causing a form of 'internal tamponade'.

One model of pulmonary circulation uses the concept of pulmonary vascular *impedance* rather than that of *resistance*. Impedance calculations allow for the effects of blood viscosity, pulsatile flow, reflected waves, and arterial compliance. Thus, the dynamic relationship between flow and pressure can be more comprehensively understood. Unfortunately, it remains difficult to obtain all the data required for this calculation, and the simpler calculations of vascular resistance are used. Nonetheless, a very important factor in calculating impedance in the pulmonary circulation is the heart rate, and for a given cardiac output, impedance is lowest at a faster heart rate, typically greater than 90 beats/min.

Conduct of anaesthesia

Severe pulmonary hypertension and incipient RV failure present some of the most challenging problems to the anaesthetist.

As with all anaesthetic plans, the nature of the planned surgery will influence the choice of technique, where appropriate regional anaesthesia may be the option of choice:

- Increases in pulmonary vascular resistance/impedance are poorly tolerated by the compromised RV, and hypertensive surges should be avoided.

- Hypoxaemia will worsen existing pulmonary hypertension.

- Correct fluid loading is critical, and monitoring strategies should include means to estimate both RV and LV filling pressures.

There are many therapeutic options to reduce PA pressure and support the failing or vulnerable RV:

- Increasing the inspired oxygen concentration.

- Speeding up the heart rate to relative tachycardia (90–120 beats/min).

- Vasodilators have a role to play, and nitroglycerine can reduce PA pressure, though often at the expense of systemic blood pressure.

- Inhaled agents such as nitric oxide and prostacycline can certainly reduce PA pressure. Although the use of inhaled nitric oxide in particular has not been universally accepted, it should be kept in mind as an option in patients with severe pulmonary hypertension and RV failure.

Inotropic drugs may be useful:

- Milrinone has specifically beneficial effects on reducing pulmonary vascular resistance, as well as being inotropic to the RV.[7]

- Dobutamine also has the potential to improve RV haemodynamics and reduce PA pressure, particularly where LV failure is a feature.

- Isoprenaline has also been used extensively in the cardiac surgical patient population to treat RV failure and pulmonary hypertension.

Further reading

Yarmush L. Noncardiac surgery in the patient with valvular heart disease. *Anesthesiol Clin North Am* 1997; **15**: 69–91.

ACC/AHA guidelines for the management of patients with valvular heart disease. A report of the American College of Cardiology/American Heart Association. Task force on practice guidelines (Committee on management of patients with valvular heart disease). *J Am Coll Cardiol* 1998; **32**: 1486–588.

Carabello BA, Crawford FA. Valvular heart disease. *N Engl J Med* 1997; **337**: 32–41.

Riedel B. The pathophysiology and management of perioperative pulmonary hypertension with specific emphasis on the period following cardiac surgery. *Int Anesthesiol Clin* 1999; **37**: 55–79.

References

1. Goldman L, Caldera DL, Nussbaum SR *et al.* Multifactorial index of cardiac risk in noncardiac surgical procedures. *N Engl J Med* 1977; **297**: 845–50.

2. O'Keefe JH, Shub C, Rettke SR. Risk of noncardiac surgical procedures in patients with aortic stenosis. *Mayo Clin Proc* 1989; **64**: 400–5.

3. Brian JE Jr, Seifen AB, Clark RB, Robertson DM, Quirk JG. Aortic stenosis, cesarean delivery, and epidural anesthesia. *J Clin Anesth* Mar–Apr 1993; **5 (2)**: 154–7.

4. Brighouse D. Anaesthesia for caesarean section in patients with aortic stenosis: the case for regional anaesthesia. *Anaesthesia* Feb 1998; **53 (2)**: 107–9.

5. Colclough GW, Ackerman WE 3rd, Walmsley PM, Hessel EA. Epidural anesthesia for a parturient with critical aortic stenosis. *J Clin Anesth* 1995; **7**: 264–5.

6. Collard CD, Eappen S, Lynch EP, Concepcion M. Continuous spinal anesthesia with invasive hemodynamic monitoring for surgical repair of the hip in two patients with severe aortic stenosis. *Anesth Analg* 1995; **81**: 195–8.

7. Chen EP, Bittner HB, Davis D, Van Trigt P. Milrinone improves pulmonary hemodynamics and right ventricular function in chronic pulmonary hypertension. *Ann Thorac Surg* 1997; **63**: 814–21.

11

EMERGENCY ABDOMINAL AORTIC SURGERY

Emergency aortic surgery is predominantly the surgery of leaking or ruptured aortic aneurysms, or of painful, rapidly expanding aneurysms:

- The incidence of abdominal aortic aneurysm is continuing to increase, especially in the western world[1] and accounts for 2% of all deaths in men over 60 years of age in the UK.

- The vast majority of abdominal aortic aneurysms are related to athero-sclerotic disease.

- Increasing incidence occurs with male sex, smoking, age, diabetes, and hypertension.

Associated morbidity is very common, mainly due to the common aetiological features. Consequently there is a high incidence of coronary artery disease, reno-vascular disease, and cerebrovascular disease. Similarly, other smoking-related diseases are common. This consequently leads to a challenging operation with a high morbidity and mortality.

Ruptured aneurysms, untreated, are universally fatal:[2]

- Even with modern surgical and anaesthetic/intensive care intervention, the overall survival rates have changed little over the last few decades.[3,4]

- Overall mortality rates of up to 90% are reported for ruptured aneurysms[5,6] in stark contrast to < 5% for elective repair.[7] About half of the deaths occur before the patient reaches hospital.[6]

In some cases of a 'leaking' (i.e. a contained bleed) or painful, rapidly expanding aneurysm, an operation better described as 'urgent' may be possible, but in general, patients present shocked and often moribund, and anaesthesia, operation and resuscitation are simultaneous and interrelated.

Despite these pessimistic figures, patients who survive the peri-operative period, appear to have good long-term survival.[5,8]

Not surprisingly, it is difficult to conduct proper scientific studies comparing different treatment strategies in this group of patients. There is a dearth of recent publications, and often personal experience and evidence at an almost anecdotal level, or that derived from, say, trauma surgery or even animal work must be extrapolated to guide one's approach.

It is known that results are better when both surgeon and anaesthetist are experienced and in current practice with this type of surgery. Whilst this is accepted, it is difficult to believe that moving a moribund patient 40 or 50 miles to benefit from this expertise (should he be fortunate enough to survive the journey) actually constitutes 'best care'. The cynics would suggest that the improved survival of regional centres is in part because the patients are pre-selected by having survived the ambulance journey! It seems likely, therefore, that emergency aortic surgery will continue to be performed in the hospital to which it presents, perhaps by a team for whom this would not normally be a part of their routine work.

ASSESSMENT AND PREPARATION

Inevitably, time is limited to assess and improve these patients. As far as possible, a history should be sought, not so much of the presenting complaint, as of general health and co-morbidity. The physiological stress of this type of surgery is very great, and, as with other major surgery, even patients who have been 'very fit for their age' seem to experience an acceleration of physiological age to reach their chronological age peri-operatively. It is known that mortality increases with age but it seems impossible to assign an absolute age of cut-off for survival. Poor prognostic signs include:[3,6,9]

- females,
- age > 75,
- actual aortic rupture,
- cardiopulmonary resuscitation (especially prior to surgery),
- hypotension (< 90 mmHg) pre- and intra-operatively (despite fluid resuscitation),
- transfusion requirements in excess of 3 l,
- raised creatinine,
- obtunded consciousness and pre-operative haemoglobin (Hb) < 10 g/dl, have also been associated with poor survival.

To these must be added the contribution of pre-existing medical problems. Ischaemic heart disease, chronic lung disease, renal insufficiency and hypertension are all common, and make the situation less hopeful. Heart failure is especially problematic.

Ideally, the decision to proceed to surgery should be an active one, taken jointly by a senior surgeon and anaesthetist, with the accent on a possible survivor rather than a last desperate throw of the die.

In practice, there is often very little time for consideration or discussion, and the anaesthetist may well be presented with a 'fait accomplis' in that the patient and relatives are expecting an operation, and are aware that survival is unlikely without. In any case, there is a large element of judgement involved, and it is natural to 'give the patient a chance' unless it is obvious (usually only in hindsight) that the patient has no realistic prospect of survival. There is often very little to go on in the way of investigations:

- Measurement of full blood count, urea and electrolytes, and blood glucose can all guide further management.

- A 12-lead ECG can give an indication of previous cardiac insults as well as present cardiac function/rhythm.

- Plain chest X-rays offer little useful information in these patients and can delay surgery.

- Blood (10 units), fresh-frozen plasma (FFP), and platelets should be requested.

- If time permits, and a peripheral pulse is palpable, an arterial blood gas analysis may give helpful information as to the true severity of the patient's condition, and, of course, it is helpful if an arterial cannula is placed to obtain the sample.

Fluid resuscitation in its own right is also controversial.[10] There is clear evidence that over zealous raising of blood pressure prior to surgery may lead to further bleeding, dislodging of haematoma and dilutional coagulopathy; in effect making matters worse. Against this is the problem of prolonged tissue ischaemia exacerbating reperfusion injuries, and renal and cardiac ischaemia. (There are similar issues involving patients with penetrating trauma which are discussed in Chapter 6.)

The controversy as to the relative benefits of colloid or crystalloid in resuscitation remains unresolved after many years of investigation. This surely means that, provided the different dynamics of the two are understood, and allowed for, it does not really matter. This issue is further discussed in Chapter 6.

CONDUCT OF ANAESTHESIA

Once the decision to operate has been taken, the patient is transferred to theatre, where resuscitation can continue simultaneous with surgical preparations. These patients are often distressed, and may be in considerable pain. Clearly, to be effective, analgesics must be given intravenously, but great care must be taken, as the patient will be exquisitely sensitive to their depressant effects. They will be reliant on abdominal tone to tamponade the aneurysm and sympathetic nervous system activity to maintain their blood pressure:

- Anaesthetists should be clear that getting the aorta cross clamped is what is going to save the patient's life.

- In a shocked patient surgery should not be delayed whilst central lines and arterial lines are placed.

- At least two wide-bore (16g or 14g) cannulae are the minimum pre-induction.

- Fluid warmers and rapid infusion devices should be available and primed.

At least two anaesthetists are required in the initial stages, allowing one to concentrate on anaesthesia and respond to the patient's rapidly changing physiology and the second to perform practical tasks such as invasive line placement when it is deemed safe to do so. At least one of the anaesthetists should be a consultant.

The patient is resuscitated and anaesthetised on the operating table. Access to radial arteries and peripheral veins will be required so the patient's arms are placed out on arm boards. Despite the urgency of the operation, attention still needs to be made to pressure area care, and vulnerable nerves. A urinary catheter should be passed, if this has not been done already, and the hourly measuring chamber brought to the head of the table, so that it can be observed easily by the anaesthetist. At some appropriate stage a nasogastric tube should be passed as the retroperitoneal haematoma invariably causes a post-operative ileus:

- Monitoring with ECG, SpO_2, NIBP is the mandatory minimum prior to induction, with gas analysis (capnography, O_2, volatile agent) and ventilatory parameters after induction.

- When practical, core temperature, invasive arterial pressures, central venous pressures and possibly pulmonary artery pressure monitoring will be required.

- Resuscitation drugs including epinephrine, vasoconstrictor agents (direct acting alpha agonist) such as metaraminol or methoxamine should be available and prepared for use.

- The surgeon should be scrubbed, with 'knife in hand' and the patient's abdomen both 'prepped' and draped prior to induction.

Temperature maintenance is important and although cooling may be said to give some protection to the vessel rich organs, the effects of hypothermia on blood clotting and metabolism more than outweigh this, so an active warm air heating blanket is placed over the patient's torso, arms and head.

Choice of anaesthetic will be a personal one (see also Chapter 6 for discussions on choice of anaesthetic agent in the shocked patient) and in reality it may be the care with which it is given that is most important:

- The guiding principle however, is to use cardiovascularly stable drugs that will produce the least impact on an already severely compromised patient.

- A 'rapid sequence' technique with cricoid pressure is mandatory. The patient may not be fasted, and even if he is, there is clearly intra-abdominal pathology that will impair gastric emptying!

- Various combinations of drugs can be used including midazolam, etomidate, ketamine, thiopentone, fentanyl or remifentanil.

- This is followed by an intubating dose of suxamethonium and intubation.

Surgery usually commences as soon as intubation is achieved. Clearly communication between anaesthetist and surgeon is essential throughout the operation, but never more so than at this point.

Maintenance of anaesthesia again follows the same principles as induction:

- Cardiostability is the primary requirement.

- Again, combinations of opiates, volatile, and benzodiazepines are frequently used together with a non-depolarising neuromuscular blocking agent.

- Ventilation with oxygen/air mixtures avoids the cardio-depressant effects of nitrous oxide on the circulation, helps prevent peripheral atelectasis, and expansion of gas spaces in the bowel. An FiO_2 of 0.5 is probably the minimum that is appropriate. The patient should be ventilated to normocapnia. This will be influenced by arterial blood gas analysis.

- Given the unpredictability of the coagulation process peri-operatively, and the de-stabilisation of the cardiovascular picture likely to be caused, the use of epidural regional blockade in the emergency context is not wise.

With the onset of anaesthesia and loss of abdominal wall tamponade, there will usually be a steep fall in blood pressure. This can be opposed by the use of fluids and vasopressors, but at this stage, the patient relies upon the rapid and effective placing of the cross-clamp to give control of the aortic bleed:

- This involves a laparotomy using either a transverse abdominal or vertical midline incision.

- The aorta and haematoma are then identified in the posterior peritoneum and the superior neck of the aneurysm clamped.

- Surgical mishaps such as aortic, or worse, caval tears can lead to a rapid demise of the patient, due to the torrential bleeding that ensures.

- Once the aorta is clamped and bleeding controlled, the blood pressure should start to come up with continued resuscitation, and the operation moves into its middle phase.

- This involves the surgeon opening or resecting the aneurysm, evacuating haematoma and by-passing the aneurysm with an artificial graft.

CROSS-CLAMP PHASE

The magnitude and significance of the haemodynamic changes caused by cross clamping are related to the level of the aorta at which the clamp is applied.[11] The reduction in effective vascular capacity causes:

- ↑ Afterload.

- ↑ Preload and pulmonary capillary wedge pressure (PCWP).

- ↑ Myocardial oxygen demand. Myocardial ischaemia is common which may respond to GTN.

- Cardiac output often falls especially in patients with coronary artery disease.

- Some of these changes, e.g. the increase in afterload may be controlled with either volatile agents or vasodilators.

- These changes may be reduced in patients who are hypovolaemic – thus the above effects may be less significant in emergency, bleeding patients than in elective aortic surgery.

High aortic clamps may result in spinal cord ischaemia. Blood supply to the thoracolumbar area of the cord is derived from the artery of Adamkiewicz – vulnerable to the 'steal' phenomenon. Prevention of this disastrous complication is helped by fast surgery and maintaining best possible cardiac function.

Renal blood flow falls with aortic cross clamping – 80% fall with suprarenal clamping but even infrarenal clamping causes falls of approximately 40%. There is no reliable way to preserve renal function (see also the chapter on Perioperative Renal Insufficiency and Failure). A short cross-clamp time is crucial but changes in renal blood flow and renal vascular resistance may persist for some time.

The cross-clamp phase usually allows the anaesthetist to stabilise the patient and prepare them for the reperfusion stage of the operation.

Although the retro- or intra-peritoneal bleed initially leads to a period of hyper-coagulability, by the time they reach theatre, the patient will invariably have a coagulopathy, in part consumptive, in part dilutional. At least 4 units of FFP and platelets early on in this stage are usually required, ideally aided by coagulation studies. The help and understanding of the blood bank is crucial to ultimate success, and they may be able to offer guidance as to appropriate component therapy. Some caution is required, because each coagulation study is a snapshot of a rapidly changing situation, which together with the 'lead time' in transporting and analysing the specimens, may require some imagination to interpret as the case unfolds. As well as guiding red cell transfusion therapy, the availability to measure Hb in theatre is much more reactive, and a useful aid to interpreting other lab results:

- Arterial and central venous access should now be achieved, if not already in place.

- Arterial blood gases analysis can give an indication of the hypoxic insult already sustained (there is often a gross metabolic acidosis). It should be understood that this represents a measure of the severity of the patient's predicament rather than a simple indication for, say, bicarbonate therapy. The aim is to improve global perfusion so that the figures improve rather than to treat the figures themselves. The situation is often much worse than expected.

- The use of a pulmonary artery flotation catheter (PAFC) is still controversial, and many would argue that the use of a properly transduced central venous line should give adequate filling pressure trend information.

- Should information on cardiac output be required, a PAFC may be the most generally available method, but the more widespread availability of non-invasive methods may ultimately prove more useable. In truth, with such an abnormal cardiovascular system, the interpretation of derived information is difficult in any case.

Unclamping the aorta

In the ideal situation, the patient will have adequate cardiac filling pressures, a reasonable arterial blood pressure (compared to their normal), be warm, perfusing their periphery, have some urine output and have an acid/base status returning towards normal.

In reality, the ideal situation is rarely even approached, and the process of removing the clamp (particularly for a straight graft) may well be difficult. Again, co-ordination and co-operation between surgical and anaesthetic teams is crucial, with adequate warning to the anaesthetist of the intention to remove the cross-clamp, and the willingness to do so progressively, or even repeatedly to re-clamp the aorta to minimise the incremental physiological effect.

The blood pressure will fall following reperfusion. In an elective case, it is realistic to aim to limit this to perhaps 20 mmHg decline in systolic pressure. In the emergency operation, falls are likely to be much greater. There are, broadly, three causes for this:

- Increased capacity/reduction in systemic vascular resistance leads, in effect, to central relative hypovolaemia. This is exacerbated by any actual hypovolaemia.

- As the tissues are reperfused, reactive hyperaemia occurs, which reduces SVR further. Several hours worth of metabolic/ischaemic products are then washed out of the stagnant lower body and returned to the circulation. Metabolic acidosis results. (Bicarbonate used to be given at this point but does not reliably prevent the falls in blood pressure.)

- This leads to an immediate fall in myocardial contractility, and a disproportionate fall in cardiac output. These products are also intimately related to the reperfusion injury, which we will discuss below.

Inotropes

The main object of inotropic support in abdominal aortic surgery is to optimise organ perfusion in the heart, kidney, brain and gut. If poor arterial blood pressure persists after volume correction, then some form of cardiac output monitoring will be required to guide therapy:

- Dopexamine, with its preferential improvement in splanchnic perfusion and inotropic effects may have a role. Unfortunately, this agent also produces vasodilatation, and the dose may be limited in the dynamic situation by falls in systolic pressure, requiring norepinephrine to offset this. It is probably too early to be sure of the role of this agent.

- Dopamine and dobutamine have both been used but tend to promote a tachycardia, and the improvement in cardiovascular variables may not be reflected by improved tissue perfusion.

TRANSFUSION ISSUES

If a 'cell saver' is used for elective aortic surgery many patients will require no autologous blood at all (although the average 'transfusion' will be between 2 and 4 units). In emergency surgery, the situation is different, and the patient will often start the operation with a low Hb (absolute loss into the retroperitoneum or the abdomen, and then by dilution as the resuscitation continues). As mentioned above, a consumptive and dilutional coagulopathy is the usual, and should be treated aggressively.

Aortic surgery is perhaps the area to which homologous blood collection and 'salvage' (by 'cell saver', or similar device) is best suited, and it is possible to avoid transfusing large volumes of 'bank blood' by use of these systems. The product from a salvage device is red cells in saline with a variable, but usually higher than normal haematocrit, suspended in crystalloid. Although helpful in ensuring a reasonable number of well-functioning red cells in the circulation, all of the plasma salvaged is lost, and the coagulopathy is likely worse than measurements of Hb or haematocrit would suggest:

- The use of clot-enhancing alginate precludes the further salvage of cells, so the timing of its first use is important.

We aim for a Hb concentration between 8.5 and 10 g/dl, since this allows reasonable oxygen content, whilst the reduction in viscosity can actually improve tissue delivery of oxygen.

REPERFUSION INJURY AND ORGAN PROTECTION

It should be understood that, even if the operation to repair an aortic aneurysm were not to result in any periods of hypotension, the vast majority of patients will have suffered a significant ischaemic injury before reaching hospital, and each hypotensive stress after this serves to compound the problem. Most anaesthetists would recognise that patients become progressively more difficult to resuscitate from each hypotensive episode, ultimately becoming refractory to all attempts (what used to be called irreversible shock):

- The ischaemic/reperfusion injury is central to this phenomenon.

- Reduced systemic perfusion due to the hypovolaemic shock and the relatively ischaemic lower part of the body all have an effect.

When the ischaemic tissues are reperfused an increasingly complex range of chemico-humoral reactions take place. This is somewhat out of the scope of this chapter but an excellent review by Gelman[11] is worth reading. Products of ischaemic/anaerobic metabolism and oxygen metabolism are released into the circulation including:

- hypoxanthine,
- oxygen free radicals,
- prostaglandins.

Micro-aggregates from the legs, endotoxins from the gut, large fluxes in the sympathetic nervous system plus the effects of neutrophils and complement activation all lead to tissue damage both immediately and in the longer term. The systemic inflammatory response syndrome (SIRS) is common. The sequelae of this will persist for many days into the post-operative period, and may ultimately compromise the patient's recovery.

Despite close study, there seem to be very few options to ameliorate this effect. In animal work, hypoxic reperfusion (i.e. reperfusing the ischaemic area with blood or clear fluid having a low oxygen content so that metabolites are cleared prior to re-oxygenation) seems to offer some benefit, but it is difficult to see how this might be achieved clinically. An alternative strategy is to attempt to 'scavenge' these harmful products before they inflict too much damage.

Mannitol:

- inhibits the ischaemia-induced neutrophil oxidative activity and consequent hyperperoxide production,[12]
- acts as a free radical scavenger,
- decreases arachidonic acid breakdown,
- helps to promote a diuresis by osmotic action.

Mannitol (0.2–0.5 g/kg), prior to reperfusion is thus frequently given. Other strategies including non-steroidal anti-inflammatory drugs (NSAIDs), allopurinol, heparin and N-acetylcysteine[13] have all been advocated at times. However, it is clear that no single metabolic pathway is exclusively responsible for reperfusion injury, and this is likely to account for the poor performance of some of these inhibitors in the emergency situation. In recent years, the role of activated neutrophils has undergone close scrutiny[14] and may ultimately result in therapeutic progress.

AFTER CARE AND ANALGESIA

- Provided the patient survives the operation, emergency patients require a period of physiological support, which can only be realistically given in an intensive care unit. Elective cases may be suitable for a high dependency unit.

- Although we aim to have our elective cases breathing spontaneously at the end of the operation, we would continue controlled ventilation in the emergency group.

The immediate post-operative period is typified by cardiovascular instability, hypothermia, risk of re-bleeding and considerable physiological disturbance. Multisystem support is frequently required due to SIRS and multiple organ failure. Patients of this age, and with the typical levels of co-existing disease that they exhibit, have little in the way of reserve, and unless they show a rapid improvement over the first and second post-operative days, tend to enter a downward spiral of worsening SIRS from which they cannot recover.

LATE MORTALITY

- It is disappointing that, despite considerable improvement in our understanding of the processes at work when an aortic aneurysm ruptures, and in the quality of the care we can offer these patients, the overall mortality for the condition remains stubbornly high.

- Death on the table, particularly following the induction of anaesthesia, is now uncommon, but this seems to have been converted into late mortality from multi-organ failure rather than into ultimate survival.

- It is very difficult to predict outcome, and we have all been surprised at patients who have survived against our expectations, as well as disappointed by those who have succumbed despite our (always guarded!!) optimism. It seems likely that the ultimate key to our management of this condition will lie in further understanding, and better control of the ischaemia/reperfusion injury and prevention of rupture by screening and early elective surgery.

Further reading

Thomson DA, Gelman S. Anesthesia for major vascular surgery. *Clin Anesthesiol* (Bailliere's best practice and research) 2000; **14**: 1–235.

References

1. Fowkes FG, Macintyre CC, Ruckley CV. Increasing incidence of aortic aneurysms in England and Wales. *Br Med J* 1989; **298**: 33–5.

2. Macgregor JC. Unoperated ruptured abdominal aortic aneurysm: a retrospective clinico-pathological study over a 10-year period. *Br J Surg* 1976; **63**: 113–16.

3. Sasaki S, Sakuma M, Samejima M *et al*. Ruptured abdominal aortic aneurysm: analysis of factors influencing surgical results in 184 patients. *J Cardiovasc Surg* 1999; **40 (3)**: 401–5.

4. Rutledge R, Oller DW, Meyer AA *et al*. A state-wide, population-based time series analysis of the outcome of ruptured abdominal aortic aneurysms. *Ann Surg* 1996; **223**: 492–502.

5. Milner Q JW, Burchett KR. Long term survival following emergency abdominal aortic aneurysm repair. *Anaesthesia* 2000; **55**: 432–5.

6. Semmens JB, Norman PE, Lawrence-Brown MM *et al*. Influence of gender on outcome from ruptured abdominal aortic aneurysm. *Br J Surg* 2000; **87 (2)**: 191–4.

7. Scott RA, Wilson NM, Ashton HA *et al*. Influence of screening on the incidence of ruptured abdominal aortic aneurysm: 5 year results of a randomised controlled study. *Br J Surg* 1995; **82**: 1066–70.

8. Hiatt JCG, Barker WF, Machleder HI *et al*. Determinants of failure in the treatment of ruptured abdominal aortic aneursym. *Arch Surg* 1984; **119**: 1264–8.

9. Urwin SC, Ridley SA. Prognostic indicators following emergency aortic aneurysm repair. *Anaesthesia* 1999; **54**: 739–44.

10. Brimacombe J, Berry A. A review of anaesthesia for ruptured aortic aneurysm with special emphasis on preclamping fluid resuscitation. *Anaesth Inten Care* 1993; **21**: 311–23.

11. Gelman S. The pathophysiology of aortic cross-clamping and unclamping. *Anaesthesiology* 1995; **82**: 1026–60.

12. Paterson I, Klausner J, Pugatch R *et al*. Non-cardiogenic pulmonary oedema after abdominal aortic aneurysm surgery. *Ann Surg* 1989; **209**: 231–6.

13. Kretzschmar M, Klein U, Palutke M *et al*. Reduction of ischaemia-reperfusion syndrome after abdominal aortic aneurysmectomy by N-acetylcysteine but not mannitol. *Acta Anaesthesiol Scand* 1996; **40 (6)**: 657–64.

14. Welbourn CR, Goldman G, Paterson IS *et al*. Pathophysiology of ischaemia reperfusion injury: central role of the neutrophil. *Br J Surg* 1991; **78**: 651–5.

12

GASTROINTESTINAL SURGERY

Gastrointestinal surgery is often high risk surgery. Anaesthesia for this surgery is a subject that is not well covered in many books published on the practice of anaesthesia. For example, the 4th edition of *Anesthesia*, the highly respected work edited by Miller, has no section devoted to Gastrointestinal Anaesthesia in the section on Subspeciality management. This is surprising considering gastrointestinal surgery makes up a large part of daily practice in district general and teaching hospitals alike. It seems to be assumed that knowledge of providing anaesthesia for the high risk gastrointestinal patient will be gleaned purely from experience gained in managing other patients. In other words, anaesthesia for gastrointestinal surgery is just 'General Anaesthesia'.

Paradoxically, certain rare conditions encountered in surgery in the abdomen, e.g. carcinoid or pheochromocytoma are well covered in standard texts and will not be covered here. Similarly, management of conditions such as acute pancreatitis, though surgical, are not commonly operated upon in most centres and are well covered in intensive care unit (ICU) textbooks. These conditions will also not be discussed in this chapter.

GASTROINTESTINAL SURGERY – THE ULTIMATE IN HIGH RISK

The general public (and many practitioners) would no doubt consider such surgery as open heart surgery as being amongst the most riskiest of surgical operations in terms of immediate and early mortality. In fact, certain relatively common gastrointestinal operations are arguably amongst the highest risk procedures performed. For example, perusal of a recent standard surgical text[1] reveals the expected operative mortality for the following operations and conditions:

Operation	Operative mortality (%)
Ca colon resection	5–10
Large bowel obstruction	10
Small bowel obstruction	30
Ca pancreas	20
Ca oesophagus	10

Many of these expected mortalities will be increased if performed as an emergency.

The lessons to be learnt are:

- Gastrointestinal surgery is high risk surgery and warrants senior input and appropriate facilities.

- With the expected mortality, palliation may be better than attempting a cure in some patients.

- The examples of good practice available from CEPOD, discussed in an earlier chapter, must be learned.

Reasons for being high risk

- Coexisting medical diseases. Many of the patients are elderly with significant medical problems.

- Type of surgery. Often long procedures with significant blood loss, fluid shifts, electrolyte and nutritional problems and significant post-operative pain.

- Abdominal surgery is associated with a profound physiological stress response.

- Emergency or elective. Many of these patients will present as urgent or emergent cases. This is well recognised to be associated with a worse outcome. Problems associated with emergency cases include less time to evaluate, investigate and treat patients.

- High incidence of hypovolaemia.

- Abdominal surgery is associated with significant respiratory embarrassment – upper abdominal more than lower.

- Many patients will suffer from pre-, peri- or post-operative sepsis. We all have a lethal dose of endotoxin contained within our gut!

GENERAL PRINCIPLES OF INTRAOPERATIVE MANAGEMENT

- Patient positioning important for surgical access for certain incisions. One should be guided by the surgeon but should not forget our responsibilities for protecting skin, joints and nerve function.

- Hypothermia is common during major intra-abdominal surgery and is directly related to the length of the procedure. Heat loss is maximal during the time that the peritoneum is open. Warmed anaesthetic gases, IV fluids and forced air warming may all be required to maintain body temperature. The adverse effects of perioperative hypothermia are discussed in the chapter on the critically ill patient in the operating theatre.

- Monitoring should be appropriate to the status of the patient. There should be a low threshold for invasive monitoring for high risk patients undergoing gastrointestinal surgery. Large fluid losses may occur including post-operative 3rd space losses (see below). CVP monitoring may be useful to guide fluid requirements after surgery.

- Large bore IV access may be required.

- Prophylactic antibiotics are required. Single dose prophylaxis may be preferable to multiple doses.

FULL STOMACH/ASPIRATION RISK

The management of a patient with a full stomach is an ongoing matter of debate in anaesthetic texts.

Current Starvation Guidelines for adults revolve around 6 h fasting from solids and 2–4 h fasting from clear liquids. In the gastrointestinal setting, many patients must be considered to have 'full stomachs':

- Emergency surgery. Pain, stress, trauma, opioids, abdominal pathology can all decrease gastric emptying. Patients are also likely to be unstarved.

- Many emergency patients may be vomiting.

- Hiatus hernia confers a recognised risk of aspiration.

- Bowel obstruction obviously is a potent source of pulmonary aspiration of gastrointestinal contents. Faecal matter is a source of severe problems if inhaled.

- All cases of peritonitis are associated with delayed gastric emptying.

Prevention is well established and includes:

- *Nasogastric (NG) tube*: Used pre-induction to empty stomach. Need not be removed prior to induction but should be left vented to air.

- *Antacids*: Consider use of non-particulate antacids. Can increase gastric volume.

- *Histamine receptor antagonists*: Effective at reducing both gastric volume and acidity but relatively slow onset of action.

- *Prokinetic agents*: Intravenous Metoclopramide will decrease gastric volume in 15 min. Prokinetic agents are contraindicated in the presence of intestinal obstruction.

- *Proton pump blockers*: A single dose of Omeprazole given the night before surgery is inadequate but more frequent doses pre-operatively may be effective.

Although prevention and prophylaxis are important the mainstay of prevention of aspiration is appropriate anaesthetic technique including:

- Identification of patients with difficult airways.

- Avoidance of prolonged or unnecessary airway manipulations.

- Awake fibreoptic intubation is always an alternative but has not achieved widespread popularity in the UK.

- Cricoid pressure. Properly applied cricoid pressure is the mainstay of protection against aspiration during induction of anaesthesia. Care should be taken as improperly applied pressure may obstruct laryngoscopy.

ANAESTHETIC FACTORS

There are three main areas of controversy

1. *Nitrous oxide.* Nitrous oxide is highly soluble – 34 times as soluble as nitrogen. Thus during anaesthesia nitrous oxide rapidly enters gas filled spaces including the bowel. This may cause problems with bowel distension and, after prolonged surgery, restrict abdominal closure and contribute to intra-abdominal hypertension. In obstruction, the increase in intraluminal pressure could precipitate perforation. However, in the only study to examine this issue patients receiving nitrous oxide had no increase in bowel distension or post-operative bowel function.[2]

   The increase in intraluminal gas is said to increase the incidence of post-operative nausea and vomiting but studies show conflicting results.

2. *Epidural analgesia.* Post-operative ileus involves sympathetic and parasympathetic pathways. These can be blocked by epidural analgesia leading to a reduction in the incidence of ileus following abdominal surgery.[3] The bowel is relatively contracted – which some surgeons dislike.

   Post-operative nitrogen balance after bowel surgery is improved by extradural anaesthesia.[4] Other benefits of epidurals are discussed in the chapter on regional anaesthesia.

3. *Opioids.* Morphine has a major effect on bowel motility, significantly prolonging the time for recovery of bowel function after colonic surgery.[5] Pethidine is said to cause less spasm of the sphincter of Oddi than morphine so may be preferred in biliary colic.

The anaesthetist and the anastomosis

Surgeons are often concerned that the increase in intestinal motility with epidurals may increase the incidence of anastomotic breakdown. However, a review of 12 trials has found no evidence of harmful effect[6] (but concluded that larger studies are needed for a definitive answer). In fact, by increasing intestinal blood flow one might expect epidural anaesthesia to have a favourable effect on a bowel anastomosis. In retrospective studies in Australia, death rates and anastomotic leakages were less in groups of patients receiving post-operative epidural infusions of local anaesthetics.[7]

Neostigmine increases intraluminal pressure (not prevented by atropine) and has been implicated in the past (mainly by surgeons) as a cause of anastomotic breakdown. Animal studies do not support this assumption. A large patient study found no difference in the rate of anastomotic leakage with or without neostigmine.[8]

Surgical factors are undoubtedly more important than anaesthetic factors in determining the fate of the anastomosis:

- The site of anastomosis is important – 25% leakage in low anterior resection anastomoses.

- The skill and experience of the surgeon are crucial.

- Tension on the anastomosis.

- Intra-abdominal infection is a major factor.

- Preservation of blood supply to the gut.

- No difference between staples and hand sutured anastomoses.[9]

Anaesthetists can help by maintaining good oxygenation (including into the post-operative period), prompt treatment of hypovolaemia and hypotension and avoiding hypocapnia.

For the last word on this subject, I quote from a recent surgical standard text:[1]

> Anastomotic dehiscence is related to two main factors: the level of the anastomosis and the surgeon.

Neither of these factors is within the control of the anaesthetist.

HYDRATION/FLUID THERAPY

Patients for major gastrointestinal surgery may well have a large fluid deficit pre-operatively and this should be assessed and treated before bringing the patient to theatre unless surgery is an emergency. If this is the case fluid resuscitation should occur in the anaesthetic room preferably prior to induction. Causes of hypo-volaemia:

- Emergency operation: May have long starvation time secondary to pathology.

- Bowel preparation: Can cause large fluid and electrolyte losses.

- Vomiting.

- Diarrhoea.

- Fistulae losses.

- '3rd Space' losses. Intraoperative handling of the tissues and bowel cause tissue oedema and fluid sequestration within the bowel. As much as 8 ml/kg/h of fluid may need to be infused intraoperatively to cover these losses. Extra fluids will also be required after surgery. The bowel oedema will contribute to intra-abdominal hypertension and compartment syndrome as discussed in the chapter on Perioperative Renal Insufficiency and Failure.

Volume loading is of benefit to gut blood flow – which is important for integrity of bowel anastomoses. One study clearly showed that fluid loading after induction of anaesthesia to a maximum Stroke Volume led to a reduction of the incidence of low pH_i (an indirect indicator of gut blood flow) from 50% to 10%.[10]

Perioperative blood transfusion

It has been widely suggested that transfusion of stored red blood cells results in immune modulation and an increase in infective complications and, even more worryingly, an increase in cancer recurrence rates. However, a large prospective trial using leukocyte depleted blood has failed to find any association between transfusion and tumour recurrence rates. However, there was still an increase in infection rates and a worse outcome.[11]

Thus, although the recurrence of the cancer may not be a significant concern there are still good reasons to limit, where possible, the transfusion of stored red blood cells. This is further dicussed in Chapter 15. Approaches to reduce peri-operative blood loss to limit the requirement for transfused blood are beyond the scope of this chapter.

NUTRITION AND NUTRITIONAL SUPPORT

Nutrition is extremely important in the surgical high risk patient. In its absence there will be:

- muscle atrophy and weakness,
- decrease in immune function,
- decrease in wound healing,
- impaired cough and respiratory function,
- gut mucosal atrophy with possible increased gut wall permeability.

The post-operative patient may be markedly catabolic with increased nitrogen losses. Many patients will also be malnourished pre-operatively especially patients with dysphagia or vomiting and patients with a catabolic illness such as malignancy or inflammatory bowel disease.

In malnourished patients pre-operative nutritional support would intuitively seem important but controlled trials have not demonstrated the expected benefits. Post-operative nutritional support is vital to minimise the negative nitrogen balance and to avoid the complications of malnutrition listed above. The enteral route is to be preferred.

Total parenteral nutrition

- Only indicated if unable to feed the patient via the enteral route.
- More expensive.
- More metabolic problems and associated with a reduced survival due to infectious complications in cancer patients receiving chemotherapy.
- Requires dedicated central venous access (with all its complications).
- Incidence of infectious complications related to the care of the site rather than the type of site e.g. tunnelled versus non-tunnelled.
- Usually adminstered as a 2.5 or 3 L 'big bag' feed with all the nutritional components mixed in pharmacy in a laminar flow cabinet under strict aseptic conditions.

A large study demonstrated an increase in infectious complications in patients undergoing major surgery who received perioperative total parenteral nutrition (TPN).[12] Guidelines suggest that pre-operative TPN is not appropriate in patients with only mild to moderate degrees of pre-operative malnutrition.[13] Post-operative TPN is only required if the patient cannot receive enteral nutrition within 7–10 days.

The most important conclusion is that short-term TPN is probably to be avoided because the benefits do not warrant the complications.

Enteral nutrition

- Supports normal gut flora.

- Possibly reduces gastrointestinal bleeding from stress ulcers.

- Decreases infectious complications in surgical patients.

- May preserve the gut barrier and prevent bacterial or endotoxin translocation.

- Reduced incidence of acalculous cholecystitis.

- Cheaper than TPN and with less metabolic and infectious complications.

Early enteral nutrition (EN) is clearly associated with improved outcome[14] (though a minority view would hold that EN is only better because TPN is worse, i.e. EN avoids the metabolic and infectious complications of TPN).

Certain new nutritional supplements may be of worth:

- Glutamine is an essential fuel for bowel mucosal cells (may protect bowel mucosa). Supplementation has been shown to lessen the negative nitrogen balance after major surgery.[15] A recent small study in ICU patients found a significant improvement in outcome in those patients who received glutamine supplements.[16]

- The idea that certain nutrients, e.g. Omega 3 fatty acids, nucleotides and, arginine in a feed (Impact) may directly stimulate the immune system is extremely exciting. Several studies of major gastrointestinal surgery have found a reduced length of stay on average, a decrease in infectious complications and less overall costs (despite the comparatively greater cost of the feed) in the group fed with this preparation.[17]

RESPIRATORY ASPECTS OF ABDOMINAL SURGERY

Respiratory function is significantly impaired after abdominal surgery, especially upper abdominal surgery. A combination of factors are involved:

- Reduced FRC.

- Pain leading to decreased cough and atelectasis. Pain is greater following upper abdominal incisions compared with lower abdominal incisions.

- Diaphragmatic dysfunction.

Patient factors may increase the incidence and severity of post-operative respiratory complications:

- Smoking.

- Obesity.

- Chronic obstructive pulmonary disease.

Anaesthetic factors:

- Most studies have examined the effects of different analgesic regimens. Meta analysis confirms that the excellent post-operative analgesia with continuous epidural analgesia leads to a reduction in respiratory complications.[18] The impairment in respiratory function following abdominal surgery is lessened – but respiratory function is still reduced compared to pre-operative values.

- Large tidal volumes during anaesthesia are beneficial on respiratory function[19] but it is less certain if there are residual benefits post-operatively. PEEP has been shown to be beneficial in morbidly obese patients but not normal patients.[20]

- Interestingly, pancuronium is associated with post-operative complications when given for patients undergoing lengthy operations compared with atracurium[21] – implying perhaps that repeated doses of pancuronium are associated with residual neuromuscular blockade.

Surgical factors:

- Surgical factors have been less well studied but it seems that length of surgery and blood loss are predictors of post-operative respiratory complications.

- Intra-abdominal sepsis leads pre-operatively to a classical rapid shallow breathing pattern and increased ventilatory demand due to increased energy expenditure with potential for post-operative problems especially if the patient's reserve is such that they cannot meet the increased demands.[22]

- A recent study has challenged some assumptions regarding the site of incision as a factor in respiratory complications. The results showed no statistically significant difference in pulmonary function, morbidity or analgesia consumption following transverse or midline abdominal incisions.[23]

Several randomised trials have demonstrated the role of physiotherapy in reducing respiratory complications following abdominal surgery. Physiotherapy is beneficial both prophylactically, i.e. pre-operatively and also post-operatively. One large study concluded that low risk patients benefit from breathing excercises and high risk patients benefit from incentive spirometry excercises.[24]

STRESS RESPONSE TO ABDOMINAL SURGERY

- The intensity of the stress response is related to the degree of tissue trauma, i.e. minor surgery stimulates a minor, transient response whereas major abdominal surgery may stimulate a stress response lasting days to even weeks. Other factors promoting the stress response after major abdominal surgery include gut stimuli via the sympathetic nervous system, local tissue factors and cytokines. Haemorrhage, hypothermia, sepsis and acidosis will all exacerbate the response.

- The response is multifactorial, thus neural blockade will not completely prevent this.

- The role of the stress response is to mobilise substrate and acute proteins for wound healing and the inflammatory response. Possible detrimental effects of a profound stress response following major surgery include increased demands on organs which may have reduced reserve, pulmonary complications, thromboembolism and pain and fatigue. The appropriateness of an unmodified response is, therefore, debatable.

- Intraoperative regional anaesthesia may only delay the development of the stress response. The optimum duration of blockade is not known.

- If the response is desired to be modified into the post-operative period a continuous regional technique is required – continuous epidural analgesia has been most studied.

- Epidural analgesia has significant modifying effects on the hormonal and catecholamine responses to lower abdominal surgery.

- The effects of epidural anaesthesia on the stress response following upper abdominal and thoracic surgery is less impressive. This could be due to failure to adequately block all afferent stimulation. For example, continuous spinal anaesthesia, with its denser block, is more effective at blocking the hormonal stress response compared with epidural anaesthesia.

- Central neural block may mitigate various aspects of post-operative morbidity but the evidence is really only convincing for decreased blood loss, reduction in DVT and limiting gastrointestinal stasis after abdominal procedures (see also chapter on Regional Anaesthesia).

- Spinal opioids have less effect on the stress response. Their effect on morbidity is unclear but is likely to be less due to lesser effects on stress response.

SURGICAL ASPECTS

Inflammatory bowel disease

Many of these patients will be very ill, pyrexial, dehydrated and septic. Nutritional state and wound healing will be poor. They may be young, have undergone abdominal surgery before and be undergoing complex, prolonged reconstructive surgery. If fistulae are present fluid, electrolyte and protein losses can be considerable. The patients have often been managed pre-operatively with steroids and immunosuppressive agents.

Perforated intra-abdominal viscus

Often elderly with coexisting medical conditions. Many will be perforations of diverticular disease or malignancies. As the presentation may be unclear many languish for several days on medical wards before presenting to the surgeons with marked sepsis. Large volumes of fluid, pus and/or faecal matter may be present in the abdominal cavity. Operative mortality is of the order of 50%.

Bowel obstruction

Large volumes of fluid may be sequestered in the dilated loops of bowel. With high obstruction the risk of aspiration at the induction of anaesthesia is marked. With prolonged obstruction perforation will occur leading to worse sepsis. Splanchnic blood flow will be reduced and inflammatory mediators released.

Percutaneous drainage of intra-abdominal abscesses

Radiological techniques for drainage of intra-abdominal collections are constantly advancing. Unfortunately there are no prospective randomised trials comparing 'open' drainage versus percutaneous drainage. Large retrospective comparisons suggest that there are no differences in morbidity and mortality.[25] Thus, it seems appropriate to prefer radiologically guided percutaneous drainage of abscesses and other collections where possible.

Empirical laparotomy in post-operative sepsis

In the face of a patient deteriorating from sepsis on ICU who has had previous gastrointestinal surgery, surgeons may come under pressure to perform an empirical or 'blind' laparotomy to rule out intra-abdominal collection. However, there is no convincing evidence to support such an approach.[26] Advances in radiological diagnosis and radiologically guided drainage of collections have reduced the place for such exploratory surgery.

Resection of perforated colon versus drainage and colostomy formation

Although technically a more demanding operation, resection of perforated colon seems preferable to drainage and colostomy formation. Several series have confirmed this to be so. Pooled data suggest lower mortality, morbidity, hospital stay and rate of fistula formation.[26]

Primary anastomosis following colonic perforation

An anastomosis at the time of initial surgery prevents ongoing morbidity from a colostomy and the need for further surgery for closure. However, standard teaching has been that anastomotic breakdown is high in the face of an inflammatory peritonitis. A recent review of pooled data from retrospective studies provide evidence that primary anastomosis is not associated with increased complications and may even be preferable.[26]

Further reading

Richardson J, Sabanathan S. Prevention of respiratory complications after abdominal surgery. *Thorax* 1997; **52 (suppl. 3)**: S35–40.

Steinbrook RA. Epidural anesthesia and gastrointestinal motility. *Anesth Analg* 1998; **86**: 837–44.

Ogilvy AJ, Smith G. The gastrointestinal tract after anaesthesia. *Eur J Anaesthesiol Suppl* 1995; **10**: 35–42.

References

1. Burnand KG, Young AE (eds), *The New Aird's Companion to Surgical Studies*. London: Churchill Livingstone, 1998.

2. Krogh B, Jorn Jensen P, Henneberg SW *et al*. Nitrous oxide does not influence operating conditions or postoperative course in colonic surgery. *Br J Anaesth* 1994; **72**: 55–7.

3. Morimoto H, Cullen JJ, Messick JM *et al*. Epidural analgesia shortens postoperative ileus after ileal pouch-anal canal anastomosis. *Am J Surg* 1995; **169**: 79–82.

4. Vedrinne C, Vedrinne JM, Guirard M, Patricot MC, Bouletreau P. Nitrogen sparing effect of epidural administration of local anaesthetics in colon surgery. *Anesth Analg* 1989; **60**: 354–9.

5. Cali RL, Meade PG, Swanson MS *et al*. Effect of morphine and incision length on bowel function after colectomy. *Dis Colon Rectum* 2000; **43**: 163–8.

6. Holte K, Kehlet H. Epidural analgesia and risk of anastomotic leakage. *Reg Anesth Pain Med* 2001; **26**: 111–17.

7. Ryan P, Schweitzer S, Collopy B *et al*. Combined epidural and general anesthesia versus general anesthesia in patients having colon and rectal anastomoses. *Acta Chir Scand Suppl* 1989; **550**: 146–9.

8. Morisot P, Loygue J, Guilmet C. Effects of postoperative decurarization with neostigmine on digestive anastomoses. *Can Anaesth Soc J* 1975; **22**: 144–8.

9. Golub R, Golub RW, Cantu R *et al*. A multivariate analysis of factors contributing to leakage of intestinal anastomoses. *J Am Coll Surg* 1997; **184**: 364–72.

10. Mythen MG, Webb AR. Perioperative plasma volume expansion reduces the incidence of gut mucosal hypoperfusion during cardiac surgery. *Arch Surg* 1995; **130**: 423–9.

11. Houbiers JG, Brand A, van de Watering LM *et al*. Randomised controlled trial comparing transfusion of leucocyte-depleted or buffy-coat-depleted blood in surgery for colorectal cancer. *Lancet* 1994; **344**: 573–8.

12. The Veterans Affairs Total Parenteral Nutrition Cooperative Study Group. Perioperative total parenteral nutrition in surgical patients. *N Engl J Med* 1991; **325**: 525–32.

13. Buzby GP. Overview of randomized clinical trials of total parenteral nutrition for malnourished surgical patients. *World J Surg* 1993; **17**: 173–7.

14. Moore FA, Feliciano DV, Andrassy RJ *et al*. Early enteral feeding, compared with parenteral reduces postoperative septic complications. The results of a meta-analysis. *Ann Surg* 1992; **216**: 172–83.

15. Morlion BJ, Stehle P, Wachtler P *et al*. Total parenteral nutrition with glutamine dipeptide after major abdominal surgery: a randomized, double-blind, controlled study. *Ann Surg* 1998; **227**: 302–8.

16. Jones C, Palmer TE, Griffiths RD. Randomized clinical outcome study of critically ill patients given glutamine-supplemented enteral nutrition. *Nutrition* 1999; **15**: 108–15.

17. Heys SD, Walker LG, Smith I *et al*. Enteral nutritional supplementation with key nutrients in patients with critical illness and cancer: a meta-analysis of randomized controlled clinical trials. *Ann Surg* 1999; **229**: 467–77.

18. Ballantyne JC, Carr DB, de Ferranti S *et al*. The comparative effects of postoperative analgesic therapies on pulmonary outcome: cumulative meta-analyses of randomized, controlled trials. *Anesth Analg* 1998; **86**: 598–612.

19. Tweed WA, Phua WT, Chong KY *et al*. Large tidal volume ventilation improves pulmonary gas exchange during lower abdominal surgery in Trendelenburg's position. *Can J Anaesth* 1991; **38**: 989–95.

20. Pelosi P, Ravagnan I, Giurati G *et al.* Positive end-expiratory pressure improves respiratory function in obese but not in normal subjects during anesthesia and paralysis. *Anesthesiology* 1999; **91**: 1221–31.

21. Pedersen T, Viby-Mogensen J, Ringsted C. Anaesthetic practice and post-operative pulmonary complications. *Acta Anaesthesiol Scand* 1992; **36**: 812–18.

22. Tulla H, Takala J, Alhava E *et al.* Breathing pattern and gas exchange in emergency and elective abdominal surgical patients. *Inten Care Med* 1995; **21**: 319–25.

23. Lacy PD, Burke PE, O'Regan M *et al.* The comparison of type of incision for transperitoneal abdominal aortic surgery based on postoperative respiratory complications and morbidity. *Eur J Vasc Surg* 1994; **8**: 52–5.

24. Hall JC, Tarala RA, Tapper J *et al.* Prevention of respiratory complications after abdominal surgery: a randomised clinical trial. *Br Med J* 1996; **312**: 148–52.

25. Bufalari A, Giustozzi G, Moggi L. Postoperative intraabdominal abscesses: percutaneous versus surgical treatment. *Acta Chir Belg* 1996; **96**: 197–200.

26. Jimenez MF, Marshall JC. Source control in the management of sepsis. *Inten Care Med* 2001; **27**: S49–62.

13

PERIOPERATIVE RENAL INSUFFICIENCY AND FAILURE

Surgery, especially major surgery, performed on high risk or very ill patients is commonly associated with a worsening of renal function. Indeed, the development of renal failure in the postoperative period is a major source of mortality. The purpose of this chapter is to review causes, pathogenesis, prevention and management of renal insufficiency and failure in surgical patients. Some of the principles and controversies of artificial renal support in the intensive care unit are briefly discussed.

DEFINITIONS

Renal insufficiency may be thought of as a worsening of renal function either in terms of reduced urine flow or an increase in urea and creatinine compared to baseline or normal values. Renal insufficiency in the postoperative period is common following major surgery. Elderly patients may also have decreased renal function and can be thought of as having renal insufficiency or reduced renal reserve. Renal insufficiency is a useful concept as it identifies patients who may be at increased risk of progressive worsening of renal function leading to renal failure.

Acute renal failure (ARF) has received many definitions in the medical literature. Unfortunately this makes comparisons of research trials difficult and meta-analysis impossible! One reason for this is that there is a continuum of renal function with progressively falling creatinine clearance.

Thus patients may present at any point from 'normal' to complete anuria/no intrinsic renal function. Different definitions focus on different points in this continuum:

Normal	Progressive renal insufficiency	Anuric/no intrinsic function

Useful clinical definitions of ARF include:

- Oliguria with urine less than 0.5 ml/kg/h. In severe oliguria the urine flow will be less than 400 ml/day.

- Rapidly rising urea or creatinine. Doubling of serum creatinine is significant in some definitions.

- Creatinine clearance less than 20 ml/min.

- Lesser degrees of oliguria or elevations of creatinine with a metabolic acidosis (excluding diabetic ketoacidosis or lactic acidosis).

ARF is often subdivided into three categories:

- Pre-renal – including true hypovolaemia following, e.g. haemorrhage but also other causes of reductions in renal blood flow (RBF), e.g. cardiac failure. Certain drugs causing vasoconstriction in the afferent arterioles also come into this category, e.g. ACE inhibitors and nonsteroidal anti-inflammatory drugs (NSAIDs).

- Renal – including all the 'medical' causes of ARF which are beyond the scope of this text but also includes tubular damage. Tubular damage (acute tubular necrosis) will follow from persistent reductions in RBF as above but also from tubular toxins such as aminoglycoside antibiotics, myoglobin and X-ray contrast medium.

- Post-renal – prolonged obstruction to any part of the urinary system will lead to ARF. Causes include enlarged prostate, stones and tumours. Prompt relief of the obstruction is essential.

Two points are worth emphasising:

1. Pre-renal causes predominate in surgical patients.

2. All patients with ARF must have post renal obstruction excluded, e.g. by abdominal ultrasound.

Urinary electrolytes

Urinary electrolytes and osmolality have been used traditionally to help distinguish pre-renal from renal ARF:

	Urinary Na	Urinary osmolality
Pre-renal	< 20	> 500
Renal	> 20	< 350

However, this is no more than a guide and cannot always be relied upon. The use of diuretics which increase Na excretion abolish the value of this investigation.

Difficulties in measurements and diagnosis

- Creatinine clearance is an inexact measure of glomerular filtration rate (GFR). Problems arise when collecting urine over 24 h especially in non-catheterised patients and, of course the result is received more than 24 h after decision is taken to perform the investigation! A collection over 2 h is probably as accurate especially in catheterised patients in whom one can be sure there is no volume missed because of residual urine in the bladder.

- Creatinine clearance can be estimated using the Cockroft formula from the serum creatinine. This is not reliable in the postoperative or critically ill patient in whom creatinine may be rising rapidly or large fluid shifts are occurring.

Potential pitfalls in diagnosis

- The kidneys have tremendous reserve. GFR can fall by 70% before creatinine will start to rise. Thus any elevation of creatinine represents renal insufficiency.

- Creatinine will be lower and rise slower in patients with reduced muscle mass.

- Urea is also used as a guide to renal function. However, will be increased in dehydration (in itself a valuable sign), following GI bleed and with high protein intake. Probably more useful as a guide to the timing of dialysis in order to avoid uraemic complications.

Despite these reservations creatinine and creatinine clearance remain the most useful measures of renal function in common clinical usage.

RENAL FAILURE IN SURGICAL AND CRITICALLY ILL PATIENTS – A SEPARATE DISEASE?

Kishen[1] makes a persuasive argument that ARF in the surgical or ICU setting is a different disease from 'medical' renal failure found in the nephrology wards. Little is known for certain about the underlying pathology as few critically ill patients ever have a renal biopsy undertaken for histological analysis. Many such patients are stated to have acute tubular necrosis but this is rarely substantiated histologically.

ARF in the critically ill is usually part of a multiple organ dysfunction syndrome and rarely an isolated single organ disease. It is often associated with sepsis, is multifactorial in aetiology (e.g. a combination of sepsis and hypovolaemia) and has a high mortality. On the other hand 'medical' ARF usually is a single organ disease, has a low mortality and often is the result of a distinct insult (e.g. autoimmune disease, drug toxicity, etc.). Surviving patients recovering from ARF in ICU usually do not require long term renal support whereas in 'medical' ARF many patients progress to chronic renal failure (CRF).

Incidence

The incidence of ARF in hospital patients is unclear owing to differences in definitions in studies performed.

- Community acquired ARF comprises only approximately 1% of all admissions to hospital.

- In one large study the incidence of hospital acquired ARF was approximately 5%. However, other studies suggest that in subgroups such as surgical and radiological patients receiving X-ray contrast media the actual incidence of 'iatrogenic' ARF may be as high as 50%.[2]

- Following cardiac arrest, 30% will develop ARF. The incidence rises with increasing duration of resuscitation and increasing doses of adrenaline administered.

- The incidence of ARF in general ICUs varies between 10% and 25% depending on the local patient populations. The majority of these are patients with surgical pathology. 'Medical' ARF is much less common. Associated risk factors include sepsis, hypotension and iatrogenic factors such as the administration of X-ray contrast and aminoglycosides. In one study hypotension was a factor in 85% of patients developing ARF on the ICU and was the sole factor in 33%.[3]

The majority of cases of ARF now occur in ICU leading some to question the role of nephrologists in the management of ARF in the ICU. However, the role of nephrologists in diagnosis and therapy of 'medical' ARF remains unquestioned.

The only systematic review into preoperative risk factors bemoaned the lack of consistency in definitions and statistical analysis and could make few firm conclusions.[4] Repeatedly studies have identified preexisting renal dysfunction, poor LV function and advanced age as the main predictors of postoperative ARF in general surgical populations.

The incidence of ARF is much higher in certain surgical settings and these constitute the high risk groups for development of ARF in the perioperative period:

Cardiac surgery

Fifteen per cent of cardiac surgery patients may experience elevations of creatinine in the postoperative period. There seems to be a linear relationship between bypass time and ARF.

With a more stringent definition of ARF a recent study of over 42 500 patients found an overall incidence of ARF of 1.1%.[5] It is important to note that ARF following cardiac surgery is a major determinant of mortality – 63.7% mortality in those patients with ARF compared to only 4.3% in whom renal function remained normal. The conclusion of this study is that ARF is independently associated with early mortality after cardiac surgery even after adjustments for comorbidity and postoperative complications.

Vascular surgery

Several studies have identified that vascular surgery and especially aortic surgery is a major risk factor for perioperative renal dysfunction. Risk factors within this group are consistent between the various studies and include:

- advanced age,

- elevated creatinine preoperatively,

- large volume of transfused blood (itself equating with length of surgery and difficulty),

- duration of aortic cross clamping,

- requirement for postoperative ventilation and/or inotropes.

It would seem that the approximate incidence of renal impairment after aortic surgery is in the order of 25% with a high mortality.

Surgery in liver disease

ARF occurs in approximately 10% of patients operated on with obstructive jaundice.

Almost 70% of patients with severe liver failure, e.g. undergoing liver transplantation develop ARF.

OTHER RISK FACTORS

- *Elderly patients* also constitute a high risk group owing to their reduced cardiorespiratory and renal reserve although figures on incidence are less certain.

- *Rhabdomyolysis*: Myoglobin from muscle breakdown precipitates out of solution and blocks the renal tubules.

- *NSAIDs*: Block the vasodilator effect of prostaglanding. A recent paper looking at the epidemiology of ARF found that NSAIDs were used in 18% compared with 11% of control patients, i.e. the link is probably important.[6]

- *Abdominal compartment syndrome*: The presence of increased intraabdominal pressure from ileus, haematoma, intraabdominal packs literally squeezes the kidney. This causes a reduction in RBF, GFR, direct compression of the renal parenchyma and increased release of ADH and aldosterone from stimulation of abdominal wall stretch receptors. In general intraabdominal pressures of 15–20 mmHg are associated with oliguria while pressures greater than 30 mmHg may be associated with anuria.

- *X-ray contrast medium*: The risk of renal dysfunction is worse if the patient is diabetic or has baseline renal dysfunction.

- *Antibiotics especially aminoglycosides*: It seems that the rate of renal cortical uptake of gentamicin is saturable, i.e. lesser side effects including renal dysfunction if the total daily dose is given once rather than in divided doses.

- *Excess use of diuretics*: May contribute to hypovolaemia.

- *ACE inhibitors*: ACE inhibitors induce ARF in renal artery stenosis. Function often improves when the ACE inhibitors are stopped. The rise in creatinine is worse if the patient is also taking diuretics.

- *Aprotinin*: There were reports of renal problems from high doses of the protease inhibitor, aprotinin, in cardiac surgery patients. However, the most recent study found no effect of aprotinin on renal function during hypothermic cardiopulmonary bypass.

- *'Medical' risk factors*: The incidence of renal dysfunction and its severity will be increased in the presence of recognised risk factors for renal dysfunction such as hypertension and diabetes mellitus. The presence of intrinsic renal disease or chronic renal failure will also obviously increase the likelihood of perioperative deterioration in renal function.

Problem with colloids?

The choice of crystalloids versus colloids for fluid resuscitation has been hotly debated for over 20 years with most reasonable practitioners accepting a role for both colloids and crystalloids depending on circumstances. Even the colloid protagonists accept that there is no firm evidence that use of colloid infusions improves measures of outcome. In recent years concerns have been raised that the overuse of colloid fluids may be associated with a worsening of renal function. This has been termed 'hyperoncotic acute renal failure'. The original reports concerned the use of dextrans (and at that time it was thought that there was either direct toxicity or accumulation in the renal tubules) but may be seen with *excess* use of all colloids especially if the patient

- has other renal risk factors,
- is dehydrated, and

- is worse with use of colloids in large volumes or high molecular weights.

The theory proposed is that the resultant high plasma colloid osmotic pressure counteracts opposing hydrostatic filtration pressure in the glomerulus.

Interestingly, small studies suggest that colloids should not be used as plasma volume expanders in brain dead organ donors or kidney transplant recipients. The function of the kidney may be at risk.

Factors involved in pathogenesis

- In high risk surgical and critically ill patients the main factors involved in pathogenesis are reductions in cardiac output, RBF and GFR.

- Hypovolaemia and haemorrhage are obviously potent mechanisms for interfering with the functioning of the kidney.

- Because cardiac output is such an important factor in ARF, cardiac risk factors also predict for perioperative renal insufficiency and development of ARF.

- Inflammatory mediators and cytokines, especially in septic patients, also reduce RBF and GFR partly through interference with prostaglandin pathways. Thus, development of surgical sepsis is an important risk factor for perioperative renal insufficiency.

Under normal circumstances a single, short insult does not result in ARF in patients with previously normal renal function. However, repeated and prolonged insults will produce renal dysfunction and if corrective measures are not taken the patient is more likely to develop ARF. A single insult may be enough to produce ARF in a 'population at risk'.

Influence of anaesthetic technique

Choice of anaesthetic technique itself is not thought to be a significant factor. Historically, volatile agents which released inorganic fluoride were a problem but this is not an issue with modern halogenated agents such as isoflurane and sevoflurane. Techniques which preserve RBF are preferable. Central neural blockade, e.g. epidural may have a beneficial effect on RBF due to the reduction in peripheral resistance provided hypotension and hypovolaemia are avoided. Conversely, cardiac output and RBF may fall with general anaesthesia. There will be much interpatient variation.

WHY THE KIDNEY IS AT RISK?

Renal problems are common in high risk surgical and critically ill patients. In addition, ARF is an early manifestation of developing multiple organ failure.

Table 13.1 – Oxygen balance in different organs (measurements in ml/min/100 g).

Organ	O$_2$ delivery	Blood flow	O$_2$ consumption	O$_2$ consumption/ delivery ratio
Kidney	84.0	420	6.8	8
Kidney medulla	7.6	190	6.0	79*
Hepatoportal	11.6	58	2.2	18
Brain	10.8	54	37	34
Muscle	0.5	2.7	0.18	34
Heart	16.8	84	11.0	65

Reproduced with permission from Brezis M, Rosen S, Epstein FH. Acute renal failure. In Brenner BM, Rector FC Jr (eds), *The Kidney*, 4th edn. Philadelphia: WB Saunders, 1991: 993–1061.

This is despite the kidney arguably being the best perfused and oxygenated organ in the body – receiving almost 25% of the total cardiac output. This high blood flow is necessary to provide the high volumes of filtrate required for removal of waste products. Despite this high blood flow the kidney is usually the first organ to fail in shock or multiple organ failure. Why is this? Why is the kidney so vulnerable that it has been referred to as the body's 'innocent bystander'?

Table 13.1 illustrates the problem and its mechanisms.

Thus although the kidney itself has a relatively low O$_2$ consumption to delivery ratio, the renal medulla (the metabolically active part of the kidney) has a very high ratio. Indeed, the highest ratio in the body. Higher than the heart, an organ anaesthetists are often preoccupied with especially regarding the possible development of ischaemia. Unfortunately, there are no symptoms or immediate signs of renal medullary ischaemia.

Kidneys are also perfusion pressure dependent. Critically ill patients especially with sepsis lose their ability to autoregulate their RBF and this becomes linear with blood pressure.

Renal defence mechanisms

Tubuloglomerular feedback (TGF) in the juxtaglomerular apparatus in the nephron is a protective mechanism which attempts to protect the kidney when perfusion is low. Efferent glomerular constriction reduces GFR to reduce the oxygen demand on the medulla. This also preserves vascular volume in hypovolaemia. The controversial role of increasing RBF versus improving perfusion pressure is discussed below.

WHAT MAY PREVENT RENAL FAILURE?

Good perioperative care and attention to detail will be the best chance of avoiding deterioration in renal function and development of renal failure.

Fluid therapy

The role of adequate fluid therapy and maintenance of blood volume as the cornerstone has been re-emphasised in a recent editorial.[7] However, proof of efficacy is often lacking. However, in certain specific situations evidence for the effectiveness of intravenous fluids has been forthcoming.

- Sodium bicarbonate in rhabdomyolysis prevents myoglobin precipitation in the renal tubules by maintaining an alkaline urine.

- X-ray contrast induced renal dysfunction. There are several randomised trials showing that IV hydration reduces the incidence of renal dysfunction associated with the administration of X-ray contrast media. Such studies are relatively easy compared to other groups of patients with renal dysfunction as the insult and its timing are relatively predictable and controllable. Although the results may not be assumed to apply to other models of renal dysfunction they are of interest. Many of these and other studies have involved crystalloid infusions usually of saline. The role of colloid infusions is questionable as discussed previously.

Oxygen transport

In high risk surgical patients the application of an aggressive strategy of maintaining cardiac output, oxygen delivery and oxygen consumption may improve outcome. One of the original randomised controlled trials (RCTs) showed that the improvement in survival was associated with a reduction in organ failures, in particular, renal failure.[8] This is not surprising when one considers the reasons discussed above as to why the kidney is at especial risk compared to other organs.

Short cross clamp time in aortic surgery

During aortic cross clamping RBF is reduced even when the clamp is applied below the origin of the renal arteries. Thus it is important to minimise the duration of aortic clamping. Once the clamp is released the reperfusion of the lower limbs will release mediators and oxygen radicals which may impair renal function.

Short bypass time in cardiac surgery

Similarly, as short a time as possible spent on cardiopulmonary bypass is important as RBF is reduced during bypass and red blood cells are damaged. Cellular debris and free haemoglobin are damaging to the kidney.

Frusemide

Animal studies clearly indicate that frusemide is protective to the kidney. Patient studies do not. Many believe that conversion of oliguric renal failure to

Table 13.2 – Mortality in non-oliguric versus oliguric renal failure.

Number of patients in study*	Non-oliguric mortality (%)	Oliguric mortality
143	28	78
462	58	65
151	42	83
109	17	52
228	42	65
125	23	63

* > 450 ml urine/24 h defined as non-oliguric. These studies were in general ARF populations. Reproduced with permission from Thadhani RI, Bonventre JV. Acute renal failure. In Lee BW, Hsu SI, Stasior DS (eds), *Quick Consult Manual of Evidence Based Medicine*. Philadelphia: Lippincott-Raven, 1997: 382–413.

non-oliguric renal failure by use of diuretics is beneficial. As summarised above in Table 13.2 the mortality rate for oliguric versus non-oliguric renal failure seems better. This does not necessarily mean that one can improve an individual patient's outcome with diuretics as there is evidence that those patients who respond to diuretics probably have less severe renal damage. Among those patients who require renal support mortality is not improved by the use of diuretics.

The use of infusions of frusemide rather than intermittent boluses may be preferable because of decreased requirement for equivalent effect, improved response and less tolerance with few adverse effects.

Mannitol

The osmotic diuretic mannitol is widely used to promote urine flow. Suggested mechanisms include its osmotic action with greater washout of solutes, plasma volume expansion and increased RBF. Animal studies suggest improved renal function but patient studies especially in the high risk surgical patient are less convincing. Many studies demonstrate increased urine volumes but are less convincing in terms of preservation of renal function.

Mannitol (in conjunction with bicarbonate) seems beneficial in the special situation of rhabdomyolysis. However, IV hydration is superior to hydration plus either mannitol or frusemide in X-ray contrast induced renal dysfunction.[9]

Dopexamine

Dopexamine is a relatively new addition to the debate on perioperative renal protection. Its actions on dopaminergic receptors undoubtedly increase RBF and creatinine clearance in animal studies and volunteers but its role and efficacy in prevention of renal failure in critically ill patients is less established. Studies in cardiac surgery and vascular surgery patients indicate some protective effect. Dopexamine may have other beneficial effects in the high risk surgical patient:

- Reduces the usual increase in gut permeability after cardiac surgery.

- May have specific anti-inflammatory actions in surgical patients.

Charing Cross protocol

A protocol developed at Charing Cross hospital in the 1990s has been claimed to dramatically reduce the need for haemofiltration in ARF in ICU patients. There are three main aspects of this protocol which, in truth, just restate many of the principles already described:

1. Achieving normovolaemia with monitoring guided by pulmonary artery catheter and echocardiographic measures of preload. GTN infusions are also used to encourage vasodilation and to reduce myocardial ischaemia.

2. Achieving normotension (for the patient's age) with emphasis on the role of noradrenaline.

3. Reducing oxygen consumption in the renal medulla with low dose infusions of frusemide.

Although theoretically attractive, widely followed and (anecdotally) often very effective this protocol has never been validated by large RCTs.

RBF VERSUS PERFUSION PRESSURE

- Many of our therapies aimed at improving urine production and renal function do so, we presume, by improving RBF. Unfortunately the relationship between RBF and GFR is complex, varies from patient to patient and is poorly understood. Thus dopamine, dopexamine and dobutamine, all widely used for this purpose, may have inconsistent effects clinically. The optimisation of cardiac output and oxygen transport as mentioned above presumably acts in this context by increasing RBF.

- The 'downside' of increasing RBF is that this presents more solute for clearance with the requirement for increased Na reabsorption in the medulla and increased medullary oxygen consumption. It has even been suggested that the oliguria resulting from reductions in RBF protects the kidney by reducing medullary oxygen consumption!

- Conversely, increasing blood pressure improves renal perfusion pressure and may improve GFR.[10] Thus increasing blood pressure with noradrenaline (norepinephrine) may improve creatinine clearance.

For example, there are numerous studies of septic shock demonstrating increased urine flow and creatinine clearance in patients treated with the addition of noradrenaline to standard therapies. The caveats are that cardiac output and RBF must be maintained (necessitating monitoring of cardiac output) and hypovolaemia prevented. The 'Charing Cross' protocol involves as one of its key elements the judicious use of noradrenaline.

The above may seem confusing but unfortunately many of the controversies and apparent contradictions remain unresolved.

WHAT MAY NOT PREVENT RENAL FAILURE?

Diuretics – the dual edged sword

The maintenance of urine flow does seem to exert some preservative effect on renal function – at least in certain subgroups such as patients at high risk of X–ray contrast medium induced renal failure. However, aggressive hydration of these patients has been shown to exert a better protective effect than hydration plus diuretics.[9] In general patients do not go into ARF because they are lacking in frusemide! The diuresis produced may be harmful by giving a false sense of security and by exacerbating any preexisting hypovolaemia.

Dopamine – its hard to keep this drug down

Despite more than 20 years of experience and clinical trials the use of 'renal dose dopamine' is still dogged with controversy. Dopamine is still widely used, at low rates of infusion, as agent to protect the kidney and prevent renal failure. This is despite numerous editorials and review articles stating that there is no renal protective effect of dopamine.

Dopamine has been claimed to exhibit different effects depending on the infusion rate:

- 0.5–3 μg/kg/min – dopaminergic effect increasing RBF
- > 3 μg/kg/min – β1 effect increasing cardiac output
- > 7 μg/kg/min – increasing α1 effect leading to vasoconstriction.

This itself represents a realisation that vasoconstriction occurs at lesser doses than was originally believed, i.e. older texts refer to vasoconstriction occurring at > 15 μg/kg/min.

The so–called renal dose and effects of increasing dosage described in the text books have always been suspected to be less predictable in the real world. Sure enough it has now been demonstrated in volunteers that plasma levels of dopamine vary widely for identical infusion rates in terms of μg/kg/min.[11]

Critically ill patients would be presumed to be even more varied in their drug disposition and metabolism. Thus there is now no real justification to think of one dose of dopamine as being a 'renal dose':

- In volunteers dopamine infusions lead to increased RBF, urine production and creatinine clearance. Animal studies suggest a beneficial effect on renal function – renal protection (the holy grail of nephrology).

- There is still no convincing evidence to support the idea that the use of dopamine at low dosage prevents the development of ARF in patients.

- What few trials there are which seem to show benefit, especially for radiological contrast medium induced ARF include vigorous fluid loading as part of their protocol.

- Perioperative use of dopamine has been widespread, e.g. cardiac and aortic surgery but this is not supported by scientific evidence.

- Dopamine *does* increase urine output, mainly by a natriuretic or diuretic effect but also by a general increase in cardiac output (However dobutamine does this better due to its more predictable inotropic properties).

- A recent, large, well conducted study failed to demonstrate any benefit of low dose dopamine in critically ill patients at risk of renal failure.[12]

Many have in the past used renal dose dopamine for two reasons:

1. It may be renal protective, they just haven't been able to prove it.

2. It may not do any good but at least it does not do any harm.

Never mind this latter unusual justification for giving *any* drug, there is an increasing opinion that dopamine *is* potentially harmful due to

- tachycardia and arrhythmias,

- reversible, dose related depression of pituitary release of prolactin and depression of indices of cell mediated immunity,[13]

- the diuresis may be harmful by giving false sense of security and by exacerbating hypovolaemia,

- a recent randomised study on the use of dopamine for X-ray contrast medium induced renal failure demonstrated a harmful effect on the severity of renal failure, prolonging the course,[14]

- dopamine seems to have worse effects on the splanchnic circulation compared to a pure vasoconstrictor, noradrenaline.

EXPERIMENTAL DRUGS TO PREVENT RENAL FAILURE

Many agents have been studied in animal models as either prevention or treatment of ARF. Less of these agents have made it to clinical trials and none have convincingly been shown to be of clinical benefit:

- Atrial natriuretic peptide (ANP), endothelin antagonists and calcium channel blockers have shown most promise but further studies are needed.

- Concerns exist with some of these agents, e.g. calcium channel blockers that interaction with anaesthetics agents may produce more hypotension which may mitigate against any renal protective effect.

- Other therapies suggested by animal trials, e.g. thyroxine have not been substantiated in patient studies.

- Hypotensive complications of these agents may limit their usefulness.

- Studies have on occasion been poorly controlled with, e.g. frequent uncontrolled concomitant use of diuretics and dopamine.

- At present all these experimental drugs remain just that, experimental.

ESTABLISHED ARF

Once ARF has occurred there are no known pharmacological interventions which will reverse the process – including diuretics. The kidney will either recover or it will not (though interesting new evidence suggests that the method of supportive therapy may influence this as discussed below). Thus the mainstay of management is supportive measures both in the acute stages and later if the ARF becomes 'chronic'.

A full discussion of renal replacement techniques is beyond the scope of this text but some interesting results from recent studies will be highlighted especially as they offer some advice as to whether there are any differences in outcome between different techniques of renal support.

Indications for renal support include:

- *Uraemia*, a blood urea > 50 is an arbitrary but common guide to requirement for support. Uraemic complications may occur with higher blood urea including pericarditis and GI bleeding. Support should perhaps be instituted earlier in malnourished patients with reduced muscle mass whose urea and creatinine will rise slower.

- *Severe acidosis*.

- *Hyperkalaemia*.

- *Pulmonary oedema* secondary to fluid overload in oliguric patient.

In modern critical care practice any of the above should be sufficient to trigger renal support unless there are definite contraindications to its provision.

Recent studies examining the role of early versus late intervention in terms of providing renal support are of interest. For example:

- Early initiation of continuous venovenous haemofiltration (CVVH) in a small study of patients with septic shock has been shown to improve haemodynamic and metabolic responses and improve survival.[15]

- Early haemofiltration is associated with better than predicted survival in ARF after cardiac surgery.[16]

- Despite similarities in injury severity and risk of developing renal failure, survival was increased in the early filtration group in a retrospective review of 100 trauma patients.[17]

Thus, many ICUs institute support at an early stage before biochemical decompensation occurs.

Continuous versus intermittent replacement therapies

A majority of modern ICUs offer continuous renal support usually CVVH. Some still offer only intermittent dialysis with some units offering both or neither. The advantages of CVVH include:

- 'Gentler'. The fluid shifts are gradual and continuous leading to greater haemodynamic stability.

- Gradual removal of solutes avoiding the potential for disequilibrium syndrome.

- Experimental role in removing inflammatory mediators in sepsis and pancreatitis.

Recent studies provide evidence that CVVH is better than intermittent dialysis:

- The rapid fluid shifts and haemodynamic upset associated with dialysis are associated with further ischaemic insults to the kidney in animals.

- Creatinine clearance falls after dialysis! (but does not after CVVH) – presumably because of these shifts.[18]

- CT studies of the brain demonstrate changes after dialysis consistent with increased brain water which are not present after CVVH.[19]

- A RCT has shown that intrinsic renal function among survivors of ARF recovers to a predetermined level in over 90% of patients treated with CVVH but in only 59% of patients treated with dialysis (i.e. more patients will require chronic renal support when ARF is managed with intermittent dialysis).[20]

- Several studies support the observation that the duration of ARF is less when the patient is managed with CVVH than with dialysis.

- Meta-analysis of (mainly) retrospective studies show improved survival with continuous techniques. Large RCTs are awaited.

High volume haemofiltration?

The volume of ultrafiltrate may be important. Large volumes of ultrafiltrate (high volume or 'aggressive' CVVH) increase creatinine clearance and may remove greater quantities of inflammatory mediators. The only large RCT of over 400 patients demonstrated improved survival with high volumes of ultrafiltrate compared to lower volumes.[21] The authors recommend ultrafiltrate volumes of at least 35 ml/kg/h.

OUTCOME OF ARF

- 'Medical' renal failure has a better outcome than 'surgical' ARF or ARF in the critically ill patient. One study from 1997 found a 16% mortality in the 'nephrotoxic' group compared to a 30% mortality in the 'ischaemic' group.[22]

- Many studies have found the mortality of ARF in the ICU to be approximately 40–70%. When ARF is associated with the need for IPPV (i.e. part of the multiple organ failure syndrome) the mortality is of the order of 70%.

- Mortality is high when the onset of ARF is late in the course of a critical illness, i.e. a recent French multicentre trial of over 1000 patients found that mortality was worse in patients developing ARF in ICU compared to patients admitted to ICU with ARF.[23]

- There is cause for optimism, however, from the studies quoted above comparing the relatively newer technique of CVVH with dialysis. In addition comparisons of different cohorts treated for ARF at the Mayo Clinic have been published:[24]

	Patients	Survival (%)
1977–79	71	32
1991–92	71	52

There was a poor prognosis if sepsis and the requirement for IPPV were combined but overall this suggests an improving prognosis for ARF.

- In addition a recent study of over 300 patients from Holland managed with high volume CVVH had a mortality of 33% compared with a predicted mortality of 67% given by the Madrid ARF score.[25]

However, it is still better to prevent ARF in the high risk surgical patient than to treat it.

Further reading

Bellomo R, Ronco C (eds), *Acute Renal Failure in the Critically Ill*. Berlin: Springer Verlag, 1995.

Galley HF (ed.), *Critical Care Focus 1: Renal Failure*. BMJ Books, 1999.

References

1. Kishen R. Acute renal failure. In McConachie I (ed.), *Handbook of ICU Therapy*. London: Greenwich Medical Media, 1999: 161–72.

2. Hou SH, Bushinsky DA, Wish JB *et al.* Hospital acquired renal insufficiency: a prospective study. *Am J Med* 1983; **74**: 243–8.

3. Menash PL, Ross SA, Gottlieb JE. Acquired renal failure in critically ill patients. *Crit Care Med* 1988; **16**: 1106–9.

4. Novis BK, Roizen MF, Aronson S, Thisted RA. Association of preoperative risk factors with postoperative acute renal failure. *Anesth Analg* 1994; **78**: 143–9.

5. Chertow GM, Levy EM, Hammermeister KE. Independent association between acute renal failure and mortality following cardiac surgery. *Am J Med* 1998; **104**: 343–8.

6. Griffin MR, Yared A, Ray WA. Nonsteroidal antiinflammatory drugs and acute renal failure in elderly persons. *Am J Epidemiol* 2000; **151**: 488–96.

7. O'Leary MJ, Bihari DJ. Preventing renal failure in the critically ill. *Br Med J* 2001; **322**: 1437–9

8. Shoemaker WC, Appel PL, Kram HB *et al.* Prospective trial of supranormal values of survivors as therapeutic goals in high-risk surgical patients. *Chest* 1988; **94**: 1176–86.

9. Solomon R, Werner C, Mann D *et al.* Effects of saline, mannitol, and furosemide to prevent acute decreases in renal function induced by radiocontrast agents. *N Engl J Med* 1994; **331**: 1416–20.

10. Hoogenberg K, Girbes ARJ. The use of dopamine and norepinephrine in ICU patients with special reference to renal function. *Care Crit Ill* 2000; **16**: 174–9.

11. Macgregor DA, Smith TE, Prielipp RC *et al.* Pharmacokinetics of dopamine in healthy male subjects. *Anesthesiology* 2000; **92**: 338–46.

12. Bellomo R, Chapman M, Finfer S *et al.* Low-dose dopamine in patients with early renal dysfunction: a placebo controlled randomised trial. *Lancet* 2000; **356**: 2112–13.

13. Bailey AR, Burchett KR. Effect of low-dose dopamine on serum concentrations of prolactin in critically ill patients. *Br J Anaesth* 1997; **78**: 97–9.

14. Abizaid AS, Clark CE, Mintz GS *et al.* Effects of dopamine and aminophylline on contrast-induced acute renal failure after coronary angioplasty in patients with preexisting renal insufficiency. *Am J Cardiol* 1999; **83**: 260–3.

15. Honore PM, Jamez J, Wauthier M *et al.* Prospective evaluation of short-term, high-volume isovolemic hemofiltration on the hemodynamic course and outcome in patients with intractable circulatory failure resulting from septic shock. *Crit Care Med* 2000; **28**: 3581–7.

16. Bent P, Tan HK, Bellomo R *et al.* Early and intensive continuous hemofiltration for severe renal failure after cardiac surgery. *Ann Thorac Surg* 2001; **71**: 832–7.

17. Gettings LG, Reynolds HN, Scalea T. Outcome in post-traumatic acute renal failure when continuous renal replacement therapy is applied early vs. late. *Inten Care Med* 1999; **25**: 805–13.

18. Manns M, Sigler MH, Teehan BP. Intradialytic renal hemodynamics: potential consequences for the management of the patient with acute renal failure. *Nephrol Dial Transplant* 1997; **12**: 870–2.

19. Ronco C, Bellomo R, Brendolan A *et al.* Brain density changes during renal replacement in critically ill patients with acute renal failure. Continuous hemofiltration versus intermittent hemodialysis. *J Nephrol* 1999; **12**: 173–8.

20. Mehta R, McDonald B, Gabbai F *et al.* Acute renal failure in the ICU: results from a randomised multicentre trial. *Am J Soc Nephrol* 1996; **5**: 7.

21. Ronco C, Bellomo R, Homel P *et al.* Effects of different doses in continuous veno-venous haemofiltration on outcomes of acute renal failure: a prospective randomised trial. *Lancet* 2000; **356**: 26–30.

22. Weisberg LS, Allgren RL, Genter FC *et al.* Cause of acute tubular necrosis affects its prognosis. The Auriculin Anaritide Acute Renal Failure Study Group. *Arch Intern Med* 1997; **157**: 1833–8.

23. Guerin C, Girard R, Selli Jean-Marc *et al.* Initial versus delayed acute renal failure in the Intensive Care Unit. *Am J Respir Crit Care Med* 2000; **161**: 872–9.

24. McCarthy JT. Prognosis of patients with acute renal failure in the intensive-care unit: a tale of two eras. *Mayo Clin Proc* 1996; **71**: 117–26.

25. Oudemans-van Straaten HM, Bosman RJ, van der Spoel JL *et al.* Outcome of critically ill patients treated with intermittent high volume hemofiltration: a prospective cohort analysis. *Inten Care Med* 1999; **25**: 814–21.

14

THE ROLE OF THE CARDIOLOGY CONSULT

This chapter provides a cardiological perspective on the high-risk patient. Most anaesthetists have extensive experience of anaesthetising patients with cardiac disease. However, cardiologists can be a valuable ally to even the most senior anaesthetist. It is important when requesting a cardiology consult to avoid vague requests for evaluation of fitness for anaesthesia. The cardiologist can be most helpful when asked specific questions regarding specific issues.

Consultation with a cardiologist may be sought to clarify cardiovascular risk or prognosis prior to a non-cardiac procedure and, consequent to that, perform diagnostic tests, review or suggest specific management options and provide surveillance post-operatively.

PRE-OPERATIVE EVALUATION

In order to identify which patients are most likely to benefit from investigation and treatment, cardiologists have sought to risk stratify patients for peri-operative cardiac complications using a combination of clinical criteria and investigation.

Cardiac surgical risk is a function of

- patient-specific factors,
- surgical-procedure-specific factors.

Patient-specific factors

The basic clinical evaluation obtained by history, physical examination and review of the electrocardiograph (ECG) usually provides sufficient data to estimate cardiac risk. *Cardiac risk* is defined as the combined incidence of cardiac death and non-fatal myocardial infarction. The history can be used to determine the patient's functional capacity. An assessment of an individual's capacity to perform a spectrum of common daily tasks has been shown to correlate well with maximum oxygen uptake by treadmill testing.[1]

Clinical predictors of increased peri-operative risk for myocardial infarction, heart failure and death have been established based on multivariate analysis.[2-6] These factors have been divided into three categories:

1. **Major predictors** (recognised markers that mandate intensive management and may result in delay in surgery):

   - acute coronary syndrome,
   - decompensated congestive cardiac failure,
   - significant arrhythmia,
   - severe valvular disease.

2. **Intermediate predictors:**

   - mild angina pectoris,
   - prior myocardial infarction either by history or pathological Q-waves,
   - compensated or prior history of cardiac failure,
   - diabetes mellitus.

3. **Minor predictors** (recognised markers of cardiovascular disease that have *not* been proven to independently increase peri-operative risk):

   - advanced age,
   - abnormal ECG,
   - rhythm other than sinus, e.g. atrial fibrillation,
   - low functional capacity,
   - history of stroke,
   - uncontrolled systemic hypertension.

FURTHER CARDIAC TESTING PRIOR TO NON-CARDIAC SURGERY[6]

The decision to recommend further non-invasive testing or invasive testing for the individual patient being considered for surgery ultimately becomes a balancing act between the estimated probabilities of effectiveness versus risk; in the process of further screening and treatment, the risks from the tests and treatments themselves may offset or even exceed the potential benefit of evaluation. The proposed benefit, of course, is the possibility of identifying advanced but relatively unsuspected coronary artery disease that might result in significant cardiac morbidity or mortality either peri-operatively or long term:

- In general, indications for further cardiac testing and treatments are the same as in the non-operative setting. *The use of both invasive and non-invasive pre-operative testing should be limited to those circumstances in which the results of such tests will clearly affect patient management.*

- If the surgery is emergent, there may be insufficient time to allow for adequate pre-operative cardiac evaluation. In this setting, post-operative risk stratification and risk factor management are probably most appropriate.

- In a patient awaiting elective surgery, who has had coronary revascularisation within the preceding 5 years and remains asymptomatic and stable, no further testing is generally indicated.

- If the patient has had a favourable recent (within 2 years) coronary evaluation and there has been no alteration in symptomatology since then, again cardiac testing is generally not indicated.

- Conversely, in the patient with evidence of an acute coronary syndrome or one of the other major clinical predictors of risk listed above, elective surgery should be deferred until the problem has been identified and treated.

- Patients with intermediate clinical predictors of clinical risk and moderate or excellent functional capacity can undergo intermediate-risk surgery with little likelihood of peri-operative death or myocardial infarction.

- Non-cardiac surgery is generally safe for patients with neither major nor intermediate predictors of clinical risk and moderate or excellent functional capacity.

- Non-invasive testing in combination with the above approach can be used to guide further peri-operative management.

NON-INVASIVE TESTING BEFORE NON-CARDIAC SURGERY
Exercise testing

The test of choice in most ambulatory patients.[7–9] Aims:

- to provide an objective measure of functional capacity,

- to identify significant myocardial ischaemia or cardiac arrhythmia,

- to estimate peri-operative cardiac risk and long-term prognosis.

Prognostic gradient of ischaemic responses during ECG-monitored stress test

- *High risk* – ischaemia induced by low-level exercise (less than 4 METs workload or heart rate less than 100 beats per minute or less than 70% of age predicted heart rate) MET-metabolic equivalent.

- *Intermediate risk* – ischaemia induced by moderate-level exercise (4–6 METs workload or 70–85% of age predicted heart rate).

- *Low risk* – no ischaemia or ischaemia induced at high-level exercise (greater than 7 METs workload or heart rate greater than 85% of age predicted heart rate).

Inadequate stress test

Inability to reach adequate target workload or heart rate response for age without an ischaemic response. In patients with abnormalities of their resting ECG such as left bundle branch block or unable to perform an adequate stress test, other techniques such as dipyridamole thallium testing and dobutamine stress echocardiography should be considered.

Myocardial perfusion imaging methods

Dipyridamole thallium-201 scintigraphy has been extensively used in pre-operative cardiac evaluation.[10,11] The negative-predictive value of a normal scan is approximately 99% for peri-operative myocardial infarction and/or cardiac death. Conversely, those with reversible perfusion defects have an increased risk of developing cardiac complications. However, because the positive-predictive value of an abnormal dipyridamole thallium-201 scan is only between 15% and 30%, other clinical variables (e.g. previous myocardial infarction, diabetes mellitus, etc.) need to be combined with the results of the perfusion scan to optimise risk stratification.

Dobutamine stress echocardiography

Predictive value of a positive test ranges from 17% to 43%. The negative-predictive value ranges from 93% to 100%.[12,13] The presence of a new wall motion abnormality is a powerful determinant of an increased risk for peri-operative events.

Resting left ventricular function

Evaluated by radionuclide angiography, echocardiography or contrast ventriculography.[14] Resting left ventricular function is not a consistent predictor of peri-operative ischaemic events. In the peri-operative phase, poor left ventricular systolic or diastolic function is mainly predictive of post-operative congestive heart failure and, in critically ill patients, death.

Ambulatory ECG monitoring

The predictive value of pre-operative ST-changes on 24–48-h ambulatory ECG for cardiac death or myocardial infarction in patients undergoing vascular and non-vascular non-cardiac surgery is similar to dipyridamole thallium imaging.[15] Ambulatory ECG cannot be performed in a significant percentage of patients because of baseline ECG abnormalities.

CORONARY ANGIOGRAPHY IN PERI-OPERATIVE EVALUATION BEFORE NON-CARDIAC SURGERY[16]

Indications

Patients with suspected or proven coronary artery disease with

- high-risk results during non-invasive testing,

- angina pectoris unresponsive to adequate medical therapy,

- most patients with unstable angina pectoris,

- non-diagnostic or equivocal non-invasive testing in high-risk patient undergoing a high-risk non-cardiac surgical procedure.

Not indicated in the following groups:

- Those unwilling to consider a subsequent coronary revascularisation procedure.

- Severe left ventricular dysfunction and the patient not a candidate for revascularisation.

- Patient is not a candidate for coronary revascularisation because of co-morbid medical illness.

- Prior technically adequate normal coronary angiogram within 5 years.

- Mild stable angina in a patient with good left ventricular function and low-risk non-invasive results.

- Asymptomatic patient after coronary revascularisation.

- Low-risk non-cardiac surgery in a patient with known coronary artery disease and low-risk results on non-invasive testing.

- Screening for coronary artery disease without appropriate non-invasive testing.

MANAGEMENT ASPECTS OF CARDIOVASCULAR CONDITIONS IN THE PERI-OPERATIVE SETTING

Coronary artery disease

Three issues need to be addressed:

- amount of myocardium in jeopardy,

- the amount of stress required to produce ischaemia,

- overall ventricular function.

Clarification of these issues is based on pre-operative history, physical examination and selected non-invasive and invasive testing as outlined above. Dependent on clinical findings and the results of investigation, the patient may require pre-operative coronary revascularisation, optimisation of medical therapy or proceed on to surgery without further delay.

Pre-operative coronary revascularisation

In patients in whom coronary revascularisation is indicated, timing of the procedure depends on the urgency of the non-cardiac surgical procedure balanced against the stability of the underlying coronary artery disease:

- Patients undergoing elective non-cardiac procedures who are found to have prognostic high-risk coronary anatomy and in whom long-term outcome would likely be improved by revascularisation should generally undergo revascularisation before a non-cardiac elective surgical procedure of high or intermediate risk.

- Patients who have previously successfully undergone coronary bypass have a low peri-operative mortality rate in association with non-cardiac procedures and the mortality rate is comparable to the surgical risk for patients who have no clinical indications of coronary artery disease.[17,18]

Indications for surgical coronary revascularisation:

- Acceptable coronary revascularisation risk and suitable viable myocardium with left main stem stenosis.

- Three-vessel coronary artery disease in conjunction with left ventricular dysfunction.

- Two-vessel disease involving severe proximal left anterior descending artery obstruction.

- Intractable coronary ischaemia despite maximal medical therapy.

Pre-operative coronary angioplasty

The role of prophylactic pre-operative coronary angioplasty in reducing untoward peri-operative cardiac complications remains incompletely defined. The indications for angioplasty in the peri-operative setting are currently the same as for the use of angioplasty in general.[19]

Following angioplasty, there is uncertainty about what should be the optimal time delay prior to proceeding on to non-cardiac surgery given the possibility of restenosis.

Medical therapy

There are very few randomised trials of medical therapy before non-cardiac surgery to prevent peri-operative cardiac complications. Drugs that have been considered include beta-blockers, nitroglycerin and calcium antagonists.

Beta-blockers

Beta-blockers should be used if they have already been required in the recent past to control symptoms of angina, symptomatic arrhythmias or hypertension. Preliminary studies suggest that appropriately administered beta-blockers reduce peri-operative ischaemia and may ultimately reduce risk of myocardial infarction or death.[20]

Nitroglycerin

Nitroglycerin has been shown to reverse myocardial ischaemia intra-operatively. High-risk patients previously on nitroglycerin who have active signs of myocardial ischaemia without hypotension should receive intra-operative nitroglycerin.[21]

Calcium antagonists

Studies with diltiazem and nifedipine have been too small to allow for definitive conclusions to be made on their use in the intra-operative setting.

Hypertension[6,22]

- Patients with hypertension have higher risks of suffering major cardiac complications during or shortly after non-cardiac operation than do patients who have always been normotensive. Most of the increased risk is because of associated coronary artery disease, left ventricular dysfunction and renal failure.

- Hypertensive patients are at a greater risk to experience labile blood pressures and hypertensive episodes during surgery and after extubation. Patients with pre-operative hypertension also appear more likely to develop intra-operative hypotension than normotensive subjects which may be related to a decrease in vascular volume.

- Patients with mild to moderate hypertension (diastolic pressures below 100 mmHg) and no evidence of serious end-organ damage should be able to tolerate general anaesthesia and major non-cardiac surgery.

- In patients with severe hypertension, particularly of recent onset it is prudent to delay elective surgery to enable evaluation of curable causes of hypertension and obtain control prior to surgery.

- Patients already on antihypertensive therapies should be continued on their medication in the peri-operative period. The withdrawal of beta-blockers and clonidine in particular may be associated with rebound effects on heart rate and/or blood pressure control.

- In emergency surgery rapid-acting agents that allow effective control in a matter of minutes or hours may be required. Beta-blockers are particularly attractive agents in this setting. Several reports have shown that introduction of pre-operative beta-blockers leads to effective modulation of severe blood pressure fluctuations and a reduction in the number and duration of peri-operative coronary ischaemic complications.

Cardiac failure[2,6,14]

Congestive heart failure is a major determinant of peri-operative risk, irrespective of the nature of the underlying cardiac disorder. The greatest risk of complications was observed in patients with a left ventricular ejection fraction of less than 35%:

- Mortality with non-cardiac surgery increases with worsening cardiac class and with the presence of pulmonary congestion.

- The peri-operative mortality is dependent on the patient's cardiovascular status at the time of operation. Therefore congestive heart failure should be adequately treated and the patient's condition stabilised for a few days prior to surgery.

- Hypovolaemia and hypokalemia are potential problems with treatment. Hypovolaemic patients are prone to experience marked hypotension during the early phases of anaesthesia.

- Digitalis can counteract the myocardial depression actions of many anaesthetic agents. It may be of value in patients with congestive heart failure, who on examination have a third heart sound. Pre-operative digitalisation because of the risk of intra-operative bradyarrythmias is not recommended except in patients whose heart failure is sufficiently severe that they would normally meet the criteria for long-term digitalisation.

Post-operative congestive cardiac failure

Usually caused by excess fluid administration; may be precipitated by myocardial ischaemia or infarction. Tends to occur soon after cessation of positive-pressure ventilation.

HYPERTROPHIC CARDIOMYOPATHY[23]

- Patients are intolerant of hypovolaemia, which may lead to both a reduction in the elevated preload needed to maintain cardiac output and an increase in the obstruction to left ventricular outflow.

- Catecholamines should be avoided because they may increase the degree of dynamic obstruction and decrease diastolic filling.

- With careful peri-, intra- and post-operative care, the risk of major cardiac complications is rare. Haemodynamic monitoring may be useful when these patients undergo major aortic, abdominal or thoracic procedures.

VALVULAR HEART DISEASE[24]

General points

- Cardiac murmurs are common in patients awaiting non-cardiac surgery. Using a combination of examination and echocardiography, the cardiologist will need to determine the underlying aetiology and significance of any documented murmur.

- Patients with valvular heart disease are subject to many potential hazards:

    - heart failure,

    - infection,

    - arrythmias,

    - embolisation.

- Patients with no or only mild limitation of activity tolerate surgery well and probably require little more than careful peri-operative care and prophylaxis for infective endocarditis.

- Those with more serious impairment of cardiac reserve tolerate major non-cardiac operations poorly, and their prognosis for surviving surgery is distinctly worse although as is the case for patients with rheumatic heart disease who face the stress of pregnancy, the risk of operation depends on the functional status of the heart.

- Patients with symptomatic critical aortic or mitral stenosis are especially prone to sudden death or acute pulmonary oedema during the peri-operative period; this may occur if demands on cardiac output are suddenly increased or if atrial fibrillation and a rapid ventricular rate are precipitated by anaesthesia or operation.

- Every effort should be made to treat heart failure pre-operatively.

- Patients with severe stenotic or regurgitant valvular disease who require an emergency operation may benefit from intra-operative haemo-dynamic monitoring, afterload reduction and preload augmentation.

Specific points

- *Aortic stenosis* – if severe and symptomatic, patients should undergo corrective valvular surgery before an elective operation. In rare instances, percutaneous balloon aortic valvuloplasty may be justified when the patient is not a candidate for valve replacement.

- *Mitral stenosis* – when stenosis is mild or moderate, adequate control of the heart rate must be ensured because the reduction in diastolic filling that accompanies tachycardia can lead to severe pulmonary congestion. When the stenosis is severe, the patient may benefit from balloon mitral valvuloplasty or open surgical repair before high-risk surgery.

- *Aortic regurgitation* – careful attention to volume control and afterload reduction is recommended.

- *Mitral regurgitation* – patients with severe mitral regurgitation benefit from afterload reduction and administration of diuretics to produce maximal haemodynamic stabilisation before high-risk surgery.

Prosthetic heart valves[24,25]

- Most patients with mechanical prosthetic valves are on oral anticoagulants to prevent thromboembolic complications. If these medications are continued through the period of non-cardiac operation, poor haemostasis, haemotoma formation and persistent post-operative bleeding may ensue.

- In patients who require minimal invasive procedures the INR should be briefly reduced to the low/sub-therapeutic range with resumption of the normal dose of anticoagulation immediately following the procedure.

- Peri-operative heparin therapy is recommended for patients in whom the risk of bleeding on oral anticoagulation is high and the risk of thromboembolism off anticoagulation is also high.

- For patients between these two extremes, physicians must assess the risk and benefit of reduced anticoagulation versus peri-operative heparin therapy.

Endocarditis prophylaxis – patients with valvular heart disease, prosthetic heart valves and those with congenital heart disease should receive prophylactic antibiotics for surgical procedures likely to be complicated by bacteraemias.[26]

CONGENITAL HEART DISEASE

Depending on the nature of the malformation, the patient with congenital heart disease may be the subject to one or more potentially serious complications:

- *Infection.*

- *Bleeding* – patients with cyanotic congenital heart disease and secondary polycythaemia are at increased risk of intra- and post-operative haemorrhage as a consequence of coagulation defects and thrombocytopaenia; the risk can be reduced with pre-operative venesection.

- *Hypoxaemia.*

- *Paradoxical embolisation* – during general anaesthesia and operation.

ARRHYTHMIAS AND CONDUCTION DEFECTS[6]

- Cardiac arrhythmias and conduction disturbances are common in the peri-operative period particularly in the elderly.

- The presence of an arrhythmia in the peri-operative setting should prompt a thorough search for underlying cardiopulmonary disease, drug toxicity, infection or metabolic derangements.

- Many cardiac arrhythmias are relatively benign. Direct antiarrhythmic therapy is often unnecessary and is usually secondary in importance to correction of the underlying cause of the arrhythmia.

- Rarely, arrhythmias because of the haemodynamic or metabolic derangements they cause, may deteriorate into more life-threatening rhythm disturbances.

- Ventricular arrhythmias, whether single premature ventricular contractions, complex ventricular ectopy, or non-sustained ventricular tachycardia usually do not require therapy except in the presence of ongoing or threatened myocardial ischaemia or moderate to severe left ventricular dysfunction when such arrhythmias represent a significant risk factor.

- Drug therapy for supraventricular arrhythmias include digoxin, calcium channel blockers, beta-blockers and amiodarone. Ventricular arrhythmias may respond to intravenous beta-blockers, lidocaine, procainamide or amiodarone.

- Electrical cardioversion should be used for supraventricular or ventricular tachyarrhythmias causing haemodynamic compromise.

CONDUCTION DEVICES

Indications for peri-operative temporary/permanent pacing[27]

- Third degree atrioventricular block associated with the following: symptomatic bradycardia, documented periods of asystole, escape rhythm less than 40 beats per minute in an awake symptom-free patient.

- Second degree atrioventricular block with symptomatic bradycardia.

- Chronic bifascicular and trifascicular block with intermittent third degree or Type-II second degree atrioventricular block.

- Sinus node dysfunction with symptomatic bradycardia.

Prophylactic pacemaker placement is not recommended for patients with intraventricular conduction delays, bifascicular block, or left bundle branch block with or without first degree atrioventricular block in the absence of a history of syncope or more advanced atrioventricular block.

In general, a prophylactic temporary pacemaker should be inserted before noncardiac operations only if the patient meets the indications for permanent pacemaker insertion **and** the surgery cannot be delayed for the time required for a permanent pacemaker insertion or the operative course is likely to be complicated by transient bacteraemia.

The patient with a permanent pacemaker

Permanent pacemakers may need to be checked for end-of-life indicators and programmed to verify normal function and the patient's level of pacemaker dependency. In patients who are totally pacemaker dependent, electrocautery poses a special problem and should be used only briefly, with the indifferent pole placed as far away from the pacemaker and heart as possible. In pacemaker-dependent patients, use of bipolar pacing will minimise the risk of electrocautery.

Implanted defibrillators or antitachycardia devices

These devices should be programmed *Off* immediately before surgery and then *On* again post-operatively to prevent unwanted discharge due to spurious signals that the device might interpret as ventricular tachycardia or ventricular fibrillation.

POST-OPERATIVE SURVEILLANCE AND THERAPY[6]

- Intra-aortic balloon counterpulsation device. Placement has been suggested as a means of reducing peri-operative cardiac risk but there is currently insufficient evidence for its prophylactic use in high-risk non-cardiac surgery.

- Intra- and post-operative use of ST-segment monitoring. Use of computerised ST-segment analysis in appropriate high-risk patients may provide increased sensitivity to detect myocardial ischaemia during the peri-operative period and may identify patients who benefit from further post-operative intervention.

- Surveillance for peri-operative myocardial infarction. Myocardial infarction occurring in the peri-operative period is often painless. In patients with known or suspected coronary artery disease undergoing surgical procedures associated with a high incidence of cardiovascular morbidity, ECGs at baseline, immediately following surgery, and daily on the first 2 days post-operatively appears to be the most cost-effective strategy. Measurement of cardiac enzymes are best reserved for patients at high risk or those who demonstrate ECG or haemodynamic evidence of cardiovascular dysfunction.

References

1. Hlatky MA, Boineau RE, Higginbotham MB et al. A brief self-administered questionnaire to determine functional capacity (the Duke Activity Status Index). Am J Cardiol 1989; **64**: 651–4.

2. Goldman L, Caldera DL, Nussbaum SR et al. Multifactorial index of cardiac risk in noncardiac surgical procedures. N Engl J Med 1977; **297**: 845–50.

3. Detsky AS, Abrams HB, McLaughlin JR et al. Predicting cardiac complications in patients undergoing non-cardiac surgery. J Gen Intern Med 1986; **1**: 211–19.

4. Mangano DT, Browner WS, Hollenberg M, London MJ, Tubau JF, Tateo IM. Association of perioperative myocardial ischemia with cardiac morbidity and mortality in men undergoing noncardiac surgery: the Study of Perioperative Ischemia Research Group. N Engl J Med 1990; **323**: 1781–8.

5. Foster ED, Davis KB, Carpenter JA, Abele S, Fray D. Risk of noncardiac operation in patients with defined coronary disease: the Coronary Artery Surgery Study (CASS) registry experience. Ann Thorac Surg 1986; **41**: 42–50.

6. Report of the American College of Cardiology/American Heart Association Task Force on practice guidelines (Committee on Perioperative Cardiovascular Evaluation for Noncardiac Surgery). Guidelines for perioperative cardiovascular evaluation for noncardiac surgery. *J Am Coll Cardiol* 1996; **27**: 910–48; *Circulation* 1996; **93**: 1278–317.

7. Guidelines for exercise testing: a report of the American College of Cardiology/American Heart Association Task Force on assessment of cardiovascular procedures (Subcommittee on Exercise Testing). *Circulation* 1997; **96 (1)**: 345–54.

8. Morris CK, Ueshima K, Kawaguchi T, Hideg A, Froelicher VF. The prognostic value of exercise capacity: a review of the literature. *Am Heart J* 1991; **122**: 1423–31.

9. Chaitman BR. The changing role of the exercise electrocardiogram as a diagnostic and prognostic test for chronic ischemic heart disease. *J Am Coll Cardiol* 1986; **8**: 1195–210.

10. Lette J, Waters D, Cerino M, Picard M, Champagne P, Lapointe J. Preoperative coronary artery disease risk stratification based on dipyridamole imaging and a simple three-step, three-segment model for patients undergoing noncardiac vascular surgery or major general surgery. *Am J Cardiol* 1992; **69**: 1553–8.

11. Ritchie JL, Bateman TM, Bonow RO *et al.* Guidelines for clinical use of cardiac radionuclide imaging: a report of the American College of Cardiology/American Heart Association Task Force on assessment of diagnostic and therapeutic cardiovascular procedures (Committee on Radionuclide Imaging). *J Am Coll Cardiol* 1995; **25**: 521–47.

12. Lane RT, Sawada SG, Segar DS *et al.* Dobutamine stress echocardiography for assessment of cardiac risk before noncardiac surgery. *Am J Cardiol* 1991; **68**: 976–7.

13. Eichelberger JP, Schwarz KQ, Black ER, Green RM, Ouriel K. Predictive value of dobutamine echocardiography just before noncardiac vascular surgery. *Am J Cardiol* 1993; **72**: 602–7.

14. Pedersen T, Kelbaek H, Munck O. Cardiopulmonary complications in high-risk surgical patients: the value of preoperative radionuclide cardiography. *Acta Anaesthesiol Scand* 1990; **34**: 183–9.

15. McPhail NV, Ruddy TD, Barber GG, Cole CW, Marois LJ, Gulenchyn KY. Cardiac risk stratification using dipyridamole myocardial perfusion imaging and ambulatory ECG monitoring prior to vascular surgery. *Eur J Vasc Surg* 1993; **7**: 151–5.

16. Guidelines for coronary angiography: a report of the American College of Cardiology/American Heart Association Task Force on assessment of diagnostic and therapeutic cardiovascular procedures (Subcommittee on Coronary Angiography). *Circulation* 1999; **99 (17)**: 2345–57.

17. Reul GJ Jr, Cooley DA, Duncan JM, Frazier OH, Ott DA, Livesay JJ, Walker WE. The effect of coronary bypass on the outcome of peripheral vascular operations in 1093 patients. *J Vasc Surg* 1986; **3**: 788–98.

18. Guidelines and indications for coronary artery bypass graft surgery: a report of the American College of Cardiology/American Heart Association Task Force on assessment of diagnostic and therapeutic cardiovascular procedures (Subcommittee on Coronary Artery Bypass Graft Surgery). *J Am Coll Cardiol* 1991; **17**: 543–89.

19. Guidelines for percutaneous transluminal coronary angioplasty: a report of the American College of Cardiology/American Heart Association Task Force on assessment of diagnostic and therapeutic cardiovascular procedures (Committee on Percutaneous Transluminal Coronary Angioplasty). *J Am Coll Cardiol* 1993; **22**: 2033–54.

20. Pasternack PF, Grossi EA, Baumann FG *et al*. Beta-blockade to decrease silent myocardial ischemia during peripheral vascular surgery. *Am J Surg* 1989; **158**: 113–16.

21. Coriat P, Daloz M, Bousseau D, Fusciardi J, Echter E, Viars P. Prevention of intraoperative myocardial ischemia during noncardiac surgery with intravenous nitroglycerin. *Anesthesiology* 1984; **61**: 193–6.

22. Prys-Roberts C. Hypertension and anesthesia – fifty years on. *Anesthesiology* 1979; **50**: 281.

23. Thompson RC, Liberthson RR, Lowenstein E. Perioperative anaesthetic risk of noncardiac surgery in hypertrophic obstructive cardiomyopathy. *JAMA* 1985; **254**: 2419–21.

24. Guidelines for the management for the patients with valvular heart disease: a report of the American College of Cardiology/American Heart Association Task Force on assessment of diagnostic and therapeutic cardiovascular procedures (Committee on the Management of Patients with Valvular Heart Disease). *Circulation* 1998; **98 (18)**: 1949–84.

25. Stein PD, Alpert JS, Copeland J, Dalen JE, Goldman S, Turpie AGG. Antithrombotic therapy in patients with mechanical and biological prosthetic heart valves. *Chest* 1992; **102 (suppl.)**: 445S–55S.

26. AHA medical/scientific statement: prevention of bacterial endocarditis. *Circulation* 1997; **96 (1)**: 358–66.

27. AHA/ACC guidelines for implantation of pacemakers and antiarrhythmia devices: a report of the American College of Cardiology/American Heart Association Task Force on assessment of diagnostic and therapeutic cardiovascular procedures (Committee on Pacemaker Implantation). *Circulation* 1998; **97 (13)**: 1325–35.

15

THE RISKS OF ANAEMIA AND BLOOD TRANSFUSION

Anaemia and consequent blood transfusion is relatively common in high-risk surgical and critically ill patients. Only recently, blood transfusion in these patients has been questioned.

OXYGEN TRANSPORT AND PHYSIOLOGICAL RESPONSE TO ANAEMIA

Whole body oxygen delivery (DO_2) is determined by the product of cardiac output (CO in l/min) and arterial blood oxygen content (CaO_2 in mg/dl):

$$DO_2 = CO \times CaO_2.$$

CaO_2 is determined primarily by the haemoglobin concentration (Hb in ml/dl) and the degree of Hb oxygen saturation (HbO_2/Hb or SaO_2, as a fraction), so that

$$CaO_2 = (Hb \times SaO_2 \times K) + (pO_2 \times 0.003),$$

where K is Huffners constant (1.34) – the O_2-carrying capacity of 1 g Hb, and pO_2 is arterial oxygen tension in mmHg.

It can easily be seen that a fall in Hb may have a profound effect on global DO_2 unless compensatory mechanisms occur. It is on this premise that red blood cells are often transfused, that is, to augment DO_2 at a time when the increased cellular oxygen demands of major surgery or critical illness put a strain on the already stressed cardiorespiratory systems so that such demands may be met:

- Experimental work suggests an optimal DO_2 at an Hb and haematocrit (Hct) of 10 g/dl and 30% respectively, above which the rheological properties of blood cause a reduction in flow and hence a decreased DO_2 overall.

- In the non-critically ill, a drop in Hb concentration results in an increase in erythropoietin (EPO) production within minutes.

- The stimulus to EPO production is a drop in arterial O_2 content (CaO_2) and so is brought about by both hypoxia and anaemia.

This EPO response appears to be blunted in the critically ill. This blunted response, together with

- decreased iron availability (transferrin saturation $<20\%$ in up to 70% of patients),

- direct inhibition of erythropoiesis by the cytokines tumour necrosis factor and interleukin-1,

- reduced folate level,

contributes to the bone marrow depression typical of critical illness.

In the normovolaemic patient, a rapid drop in Hb brings about certain compensatory changes:[1]

- **Haemodynamic** – the decrease in plasma viscosity improves peripheral blood flow and thus enhances venous return to the right atrium. An immediate increase in stroke volume follows, by the Starling principle, in response to haemodilution and is non-sympathetically mediated. The reduced viscosity also reduces afterload, which may be an important mechanism in maintaining CO in the impaired ventricle. Further, increases in CO are mediated through aortic chemoreceptors inducing sympathetically mediated increases in contractility (and so stroke volume), venomotor tone (and thus venous return) and heart rate.

- **Microcirculatory** – secondary to the increased CO is an increased organ capillary blood flow and capillary recruitment. Both of these factors are dependent upon the degree of anaemia and the individual organ concerned.

- **Oxyhaemoglobin dissociation curve (ODC)** – a rightward shift in the ODC is seen, which increases the O_2 unloading by Hb for a given blood pO_2. This is clearly advantageous in increasing cellular O_2 extraction. The primary reason for this is the increased red cell 2,3-diphosphoglycerate (2, 3-DPG) synthesis seen during anaemia. Local temperature and pH cause a rightward shift in the curve but their effect is thought to be less significant than that of 2,3-DPG.

Note: These are the responses to anaemia. When anaemia is due to acute blood losses, the physiological responses to hypovolaemia will also be triggered.

ANAEMIA AND THE HEART

Major surgery, critical illness and anaemia all place stress on the myocardium to increase CO and hence global DO_2. To do so, myocardial DO_2 must increase to meet its own increased O_2 demand (MVO_2). As normal myocardial O_2 extraction runs between 75% and 80%, any increase in MVO_2 shall be met primarily by an increase in coronary flow; that is, MVO_2 is 'flow-restricted'. In the presence of coronary artery disease, fixed coronary stenoses may prevent any increase in myocardial flow, thus limiting myocardial DO_2. Thus, during anaemia the increased MVO_2 brought about by the demands of an increased CO cannot be met, coronary blood flow is preferentially diverted to the subepicardial layers and subendocardial ischaemia or infarction ensue.

PROBLEMS ASSOCIATED WITH BLOOD TRANSFUSION

Problems such as hyperkalaemia, hypocalcaemia, metabolic acidosis, hypothermia, dilutional coagulopathy and citrate toxicity, although important, are related to massive blood transfusion only and will not be discussed further in this review.

If the purpose of a blood transfusion is to augment tissue oxygen consumption (VO_2), then certain so-called 'storage lesions' should be borne in mind as they may have a deleterious effect in this respect:

- Stored blood has reduced levels of 2,3-DPG levels causing a leftward shift in the ODC and a reduced unloading of O_2 from Hb.

- In addition, the reduced membrane deformability of red cells, brought about through their storage, is thought to impede their passage through the narrow confines of a capillary bed that would otherwise allow the passage of the more compliant cells unhindered. This may be the explanation for the observation that patients receiving old transfused red blood cells developed evidence of splanchnic ischaemia.[2]

- The high Hct of packed red cells may increase blood viscosity to an extent such that the favourable flow characteristics of anaemia are partially reversed, with a resultant decrease in tissue blood flow and capillary recruitment.

- An interesting study by Purdy[3] is the first (and only) study to report an association between increased age of transfused red blood cells and overall mortality in septic patients. The median age of blood units transfused to survivors was 17 days versus 25 days for non-survivors. This study was retrospective and therefore one should be cautious in accepting its implications, but if these findings were confirmed by a prospective randomised trial, it would have major implications for the use of stored blood in all patients.

Transmission of infection by blood transfusion

There remains an exceedingly small but real risk of infection from transfusion of stored packed red blood cells:[4]

- The risk of HIV infection is currently 1 in 4 million units transfused.

- That of hepatitis B is 1 in 100 000–400 000 units.

- Transfusion is becoming an increasingly rare cause of hepatitis C infection, possibly as a result of HIV high-risk donation exclusion together with routine antibody testing of donated blood. The current risk is 1 in 200 000 transfusions.

- Infection with Parvovirus B19 is highly variable and appears only to be significant in pregnancy.

- Bacterial contamination of stored blood is related to the length of storage and has a transmission rate of 1 per million transfusions.

- The transmission rates of *Plasmodium* and *Trypanosoma cruzi* are vanishingly small.

Immunosuppressive effects of blood transfusion[5]

The immunosuppressive effects of allogenic blood transfusion are well established:

Non-specific	Antigen-specific
Reduced natural killer cell production and activity	Increased suppressor T-cell production (high CD8 count)
Reduced CD4 helper cell production	Anti-idiotypic antibody production
Reduced monocyte/macrophage activity	
Reduced interleukin-2 (IL-2) levels	
Increased prostaglandin E_2 (PGE$_2$) levels	

Postoperative inflammatory response

Initial studies suggested that perioperative allogenic blood transfusion can induce an excessive cytokine response with significant increases in IL-6 in the transfused group. A recent study of cardiac surgery patients[6] confirmed that transfusion is associated with an increased inflammatory response especially IL-6. However, an interesting finding from this study was that the transfusion packs themselves contained increased levels of bactericidal permeability increasing protein (BPI) – a marker of neutrophil activation. Thus, the transfused blood may itself have contained the trigger for part of this inflammatory response. Further, statistical analysis suggested that transfusion was a factor in poor postoperative outcome, although a direct causal relationship was not established.

Postoperative infection

The effects of blood transfusion-induced immunosuppression have been thought to increase the risk of postoperative infection.[7,8] Much of the evidence is retrospective and not all reports have shown an effect of transfusion on postoperative infection rates. Nonetheless, it remains a possible hazard associated with transfused blood.

It should be remembered that blood transfusion is a common non-infectious cause of leucocytosis in the critically ill.[9]

Postoperative cancer recurrence

Much data exists to support the concept of increased tumour recurrence in patients who have received perioperative allogenic red cell transfusion whilst undergoing potentially curative surgery for cancers.

Vamvakas[10] disputes much of the evidence for infection and tumour recurrence, stating that most of the evidence is retrospective and that analysis of prospective, randomised, controlled trials show very little difference between those transfused and those not transfused. He suggests that differences are due to retrospective trial design and that immunomodulation occurs secondary to the variables that lead to the transfusion and not as a result of the transfusion itself. This is controversial.

Autologous or leucodepleted blood transfusion

The potential evidence for benefit (in terms of reduced complications) from leucodepleted or autologous blood is as yet inconclusive. Results are variable but most seem to support either no difference or a reduced incidence of infection and tumour recurrence with leucodepleted and autologous blood.

Blumberg and Heal[11] estimate the cost of postoperative transfusion to be on average $1000–2000 per transfusion (blood cost plus complications of transfusion). Spending $240 million on leucodepletion annually in the USA could result in savings of $6–12 billion annually whilst reducing postoperative infections and tumour recurrence rates.

Haemolytic reactions

An estimated 1 in 250 000–1 000 000 transfusions result in an overt haemolytic reaction, most commonly secondary to minor erythrocyte antigens. This is almost certainly an underestimate due to under-reporting and failure to recognise such a reaction during either surgery or the course of a critical illness at a time when the signs (hypotension, tachycardia, DIC, pyrexia) can be attributed to a more common pathology. The current mortality of 1 per million unit transfusions is attributable to ABO incompatibility as a result of clerical error in 50% of cases.

ROLE OF ANAEMIA AND TRANSFUSION IN SURGICAL MORBIDITY

- A retrospective analysis by Carson[12] demonstrated a significantly higher morbidity and mortality in surgical patients with a preoperative Hb of less than 6 g/dl. This effect was substantially more significant in patients with pre-existing cardiac disease and in those who had a larger blood loss, as might be expected.

- Other studies have shown an increased cardiac morbidity amongst anaemic surgical patients with cardiovascular disease.[13,14]

- Carson[15] found no increased mortality in 8787 surgical patients down to Hb of 8 g/dl, amongst whom the presence of cardiac disease had no bearing on outcome.

- Speiss *et al.* demonstrated a negative effect of transfusion on outcome, in patients having coronary artery bypass graft (CABG) surgery.[16] This retrospective study of 2202 patients investigated the effect of Hct values at entry to intensive care unit (ICU) post-surgery on cardiac morbidity. The risk of post-CABG MI was increased when ICU-entry Hct was either high ($>33\%$) or medium (25–33%) compared to when ICU-entry Hct was low ($<25\%$). They also demonstrated a significantly increased risk of left ventricular dysfunction and mortality in the high and medium Hct groups compared to the low Hct group.

- In a study of vascular surgery patients, Hb levels of 9 g/dl were tolerated without adverse clinical outcome.[17] Patients did not compensate for anaemia by increased myocardial work, but by increasing O_2 extraction in the peripheral tissues.

- Extreme perioperative haemodilution down to Hb of 5 g/dl in Jehovah's Witnesses has shown no decrease in VO_2.[18] In healthy volunteers, this degree of anaemia appears to be the point below which DO_2 becomes inadequate (known as the critical point of DO_2), and accumulation of lactic acid occurs as anaerobic metabolism takes over.

Transfusion seems to be commonly triggered by a certain Hb or Hct level without any evidence of impaired oxygenation of the tissues. An Hb of 10 g/dl has been traditionally accepted as the level at which Hb should be maintained. In truth, there is little objective evidence to support this approach and it seems as if this number has been chosen for little more than the fact that this is a nice round number! However, evidence already outlined above may support a more liberal 'trigger' for transfusion in those patients without cardiac disease.

BLOOD TRANSFUSION IN ICU

Studies investigating DO_2 in ICU patients suggest an ideal Hct of 33% to augment DO_2. Dietrich[19] studied the augmentation of DO_2 by red cell transfusion in volume-resuscitated, non-surgical intensive care patients. He showed neither an increase in VO_2 nor a decrease in blood lactate levels in any patient and concluded that the shock state of their patient group was not enhanced by red cell transfusion.

Impact of transfusion on outcome in ICU patients

A recent prospective, randomised study[20] compared a restrictive with a liberal transfusion strategy in 838 general ICU patients:

- Those in the restrictive strategy group were transfused at an Hb < 7 g/dl with packed red cells to maintain their Hb at 7–9 g/dl.

- Those in the liberal strategy group were transfused with packed red cells at an Hb < 10 g/dl to maintain their Hb at 10–12 g/dl.

Their results are quite striking:

- In those patients with an APACHE score less than 20 and in patients aged less than 55 years (with APACHE more or less than 20), the 30-day survival was significantly better in those randomised to the restrictive transfusion strategy.

- Amongst patients with cardiac disease, the 30-day mortality was reduced, but not significantly so, if allocated to the restrictive strategy.

- There was a significant decrease in organ dysfunction and cardiac complications in the restrictive strategy group.

It is difficult to ignore the implications of such a large and well-conducted study.

Transfusion and weaning from IPPV

- Schonhofer et al.[21] demonstrated a decreased work of breathing and decreased minute ventilation in anaemic patients with chronic obstructive airways disease (COAD) when transfused from an Hb of 8–9 g/dl to an Hb of greater than 12 g/dl. A similar effect was not seen in anaemic patients without COAD who were transfused with an identical strategy.

- This work complements case reports by the same authors concerning patients successfully weaned after transfusion to Hb greater than 12 g/dl.

However, 'difficult to wean' is a multifactorial problem for which many strategies have been employed, few with evidence to support them. Transfusion to a normal Hb in such patients remains an unproven strategy.

Erythropoietin therapy

- In view of evidence for a blunted EPO response in the critically ill, Corwin *et al.*[22] studied the transfusion requirements of critically ill patients receiving recombinant human erythropoietin (rHuEPO) using critically ill patients not receiving rHuEPO as their controls. This randomised, controlled, multicentre trial demonstrated a 45% reduction in red cell units transfused with no measured difference in adverse effects or outcome.

- Other workers have shown an increased P50 amongst cardiac surgical patients given rHuEPO.[23] This favours well in terms of oxygen transport in comparison with the reduced P50 of stored red cells.

EPO therapy is expensive and the benefits are, so far, unproven. However, if it demonstrably reduces red cell transfusion requirements and avoids the deleterious effects of transfusion, it may well be a cost-effective therapy for the critically ill patient.

PRACTICAL GUIDELINES

A major trend in recent years has been greater reluctance to expose patients to the problems associated with allogenic blood transfusion. This is achieved by:

- Many methods of reducing blood loss during surgery. These are outside the remit of this review.

- Accepting lesser Hb than previously. In particular, accepting that 10 g/dl is an arbitrary goal in many patients.

Some important principles:

- Recommendations by the ASA Task Force on blood component therapy[24] state that transfusion is 'rarely required above an Hb of 10 g/dl' and transfusion is 'almost always indicated when Hb is less than 6 g/dl'.

- The multicentre trial in Canadian ICUs would suggest that a restrictive policy (i.e. allowing Hbs to drift down to 7–8 g/dl) is safe in ICU patients and may even be superior (but further studies are needed especially on different subgroups such as neurosurgical patients).

- Many anaesthetists are applying these principles in the operating theatre and this is probably safe and appropriate for most patients. Caution should still, however, be applied in the elderly and those with cardiac disease. Few now insist that an Hb of 10 g/dl is a prerequisite for elective surgery.

- It would also be prudent not to be too willing to accept Hbs of 7–8 g/dl preoperatively for those patients whose surgery has the potential for sudden profuse blood loss.

- The ready availability of intraoperative Hb checks is to be encouraged and will permit more accurate control of blood transfusion.

Overall, the majority of practitioners are willing to accept lower Hb in high-risk surgical and other critically ill patients because of

- concerns re-safety of transfused blood,

- evidence that lower Hbs are safe and may even be beneficial,

- lack of convincing evidence of benefits of a liberal transfusion strategy.

Further reading

Supplement on perioperative anaemia. *Br J Anaesth* 1998; **81**: 1–82.

Management of anemia in the critically ill. *Crit Care Med* 2001; **29**: S139–210.

References

1. Hebert PC, Hu L, Biro G. Review of physiological response to anaemia. *Can Med Assoc J* 1997; **156 (suppl. 11)**: S27–40.

2. Marik PE, Sibbald WJ. Effect of stored-blood transfusion on oxygen delivery in patients with sepsis. *JAMA* 1993; **269**: 3024–9.

3. Purdy FR, Tweeddale MG, Merrick PM. Association of mortality with age of blood transfused in septic ICU patients. *Can J Anaesth* 1997; **44**: 1256–61.

4. British Committee for Standards in Haematology (BCSH). Blood Transfusion Task Force, Guidelines for the clinical use of red cell transfusions. *Br J Haematol* 2001; **113**: 24–31.

5. Landers DF, Hill GE, Wong KC, Fox IJ. Blood transfusion-induced immunomodulation. *Anesth Analg* 1996, **82**. 187–204.

6. Fransen E, Maessen J, Dentener M *et al.* Impact of blood transfusions on inflammatory mediator release in patients undergoing cardiac surgery. *Chest* 1999; **116**: 1233–9.

7. Murphy PJ, Connery C, Hicks GL, Blumberg N. Homologous blood transfusion as a risk factor for postoperative infection after coronary artcry bypass graft operations. *J Thorac Cardiovasc Surg* 1992; **104**: 1092–9.

8. Torchia MG, Danzinger RG. Perioperative blood transfusion and albumin administration are independent risk factors for the development of postoperative infections after colorectal surgery. *Can J Surg* 2000; **43**: 212–16.

9. Fenwick JC, Cameron M, Naiman SC *et al.* Blood transfusion as a cause of leucocytosis in critically ill patients. *Lancet* 1994; **344**: 855–6.

10. Vamvakas EC. Transfusion-associated cancer recurrence and postoperative infection: meta-analysis of randomised, controlled clinical trials. *Transfusion* 1996; **36**: 175–86.

11. Blumberg N, Heal J. Immunomodulation by blood transfusion: an evolving scientific and clinical challenge. *Am J Med* 1996; **101**: 299–308.

12. Carson JL, Duff A, Poses RM *et al.* Effect of anaemia and cardiovascular disease on surgical mortality and morbidity. *Lancet* 1996; **348**: 1055–60.

13. Hogue CW, Goodnough LT, Monk TG. Perioperative myocardial ischaemic episodes are related to haematocrit levels in patients undergoing radical prostatectomy. *Transfusion* 1998; **38**: 924–31.

14. Nelson AH, Fleischer LA, Rosenbaum SH. Relationship between postoperative anaemia and cardiac morbidity in high-risk vascular patients in the intensive care unit. *Crit Care Med* 1993; **21**: 860–6.

15. Carson JL, Duff A, Berlin J *et al.* Perioperative blood transfusion and postoperative mortality. *JAMA* 1998; **279**: 199–205.

16. Speiss BD, Ley C, Body SC *et al.* Haematocrit value on intensive care unit entry influences the frequency of Q-wave myocardial infarction after coronary artery bypass grafting. *J Thorac Cardiovasc Surg* 1998; **116**: 460–7.

17. Bush RL, Pevec WC, Holcroft JW. A prospective, randomized trial limiting perioperative red blood cell transfusions in vascular patients. *Am J Surg* 1997; **174**: 143–8.

18. Kreimeier U, Messmer K. Haemodilution in clinical surgery; state of the art 1996. *World J Surg* 1996; **20**: 1208–17.

19. Dietrich KA, Conrad SA, Hebert CA *et al.* Cardiovascular and metabolic response to red blood cell transfusion in critically ill volume-resuscitated nonsurgical patients. *Crit Care Med* 1990; **18**: 940–5.

20. Hebert PC, Wells G, Blajchman MA *et al.* A multicentre, randomised, controlled clinical trial of transfusion requirements in critical care. *N Engl J Med* 1999; **340**: 409–17.

21. Schonhofer B, Wenzel M, Geibel M, Kohler D. Blood transfusion and lung function in chronically anaemic patients with severe chronic obstructive pulmonary disease. *Crit Care Med* 1998; **26**: 1824–8.

22. Corwin HL, Gettinger A, Rodriguez RM *et al.* Efficacy of recombinant human erythropoietin in the critically ill patient: a randomised, double blind, placebo-controlled trial. *Crit Care Med* 1999; **27**: 2346–50.

23. Sowade O, Gross J *et al.* Evaluation of oxygen availability with the oxygen status algorithm in patients undergoing open heart surgery treated with Epoetin-β. *J Lab Clin Med* 1997; **129**: 97–105.

24. ASA Task Force on blood component therapy. Practice guidelines for blood component therapy. *Anesthesiology* 1996; **84**: 732–47.

16

ADMISSION CRITERIA FOR HDU AND ICU

The provision of intensive care unit (ICU) and high dependency unit (HDU) facilities is an important consideration in patient care in acute service hospitals:

- The recommendation for provision of ICU beds in the UK is 1–2%.

- In 1988 the Association of Anaesthetists of Great Britain and Ireland (AAGBI) identified 55 hospitals with a designated HDU.

- An updated study in 1992/1993 identified only 39 hospitals with an HDU.[1]

- In 1991, the AAGBI concluded that an intermediate level of acute care between that provided on an ICU and general ward would be necessary.

- In the previous year, the Intensive Care Society of Great Britain suggested that critical care should be viewed as a spectrum ranging from the recovery room, moving through the HDU and culminating in the ICU.

The development of intensive care and high dependency care has been driven by the perception that severely ill patients may benefit from a greater intensity of medical and nursing care than is usually available at general ward level. The weight of clinical opinion supports the view that intensive care improves the survival of critically ill patients (or those at risk of becoming critically ill). The distinction between a patient requiring ICU and a patient requiring HDU is complex.

Recent proposals by the Department of Health[2] recommend that the existing division into high dependency and intensive care based on beds should be replaced by a classification that focuses on the level of care that individual patients need, regardless of location.

They suggest the following levels of care:

Level 0   Patients whose needs can be met through normal ward care in an acute hospital.

Level 1   Patients at risk of their condition deteriorating, or those recently relocated from higher levels of care, whose needs can be met on an acute ward with additional advice and support from the critical care team.

Level 2   Patients requiring more detailed observation or intervention including support for a single failing organ system or post-operative care and those 'stepping down' from higher levels of care.

Level 3   Patients requiring advanced respiratory support alone or basic respiratory support together with support of at least two organ systems. This level includes all complex patients requiring support for multi-organ failure.

The review recommends that all acute hospitals carrying out elective surgery must be able to provide level 2 care. They should either have level 3 care available on site or they should have protocols in place to arrange suitable transfer. Hospitals admitting emergencies should normally have all levels of care available, although in a limited number of cases, protocols may be agreed for safe transfer to an adjacent hospital for level 3 care.

One of the important uses of an HDU is its role as a 'halfway house' between the general ward and the ICU. This means that it would provide a service for the care of patients who have improved after a stay in the ICU but who are not yet well enough to be transferred back to the ward. Furthermore, an HDU provides a halfway stage for those patients who may subsequently need ICU treatment following clinical deterioration on the general ward. Early intervention and provision of HDU facilities may prevent subsequent ICU admission or favourably influence length of stay in hospital, long-term prognosis, and ultimate survival:

- On a general ward in a hospital without a HDU, up to 13.5% of patients may benefit from high dependency care.[3]

- Many such patients are consequently treated on the ICU, so fuelling the demand for intensive care services.

- Research also suggests that establishing an intermediate level of care reduces ward mortality rates by 25% and cardiac arrests by 39%.[4]

The availability of an HDU will thus optimise patient care by

- maintaining the quality of critical care,

- protecting ICU beds for those who need them,

- improving the care of patients otherwise treated on general wards,

- improving post-operative pain relief,

- allowing a more cost-effective use of available resources.

DIFFERENCES BETWEEN ICU AND HDU

'Graduated patient care' is a concept which allows stratification of patients according to clinical dependency into those who

- should be admitted to an ICU for the management of single or multiple organ failure,

- should best be treated in a HDU.

Intensive care appropriate for	High dependency care appropriate for
Patients requiring or likely to require advanced respiratory support alone.	Patients requiring support for a single failing organ system, but excluding those needing advanced respiratory support.
Patients requiring support of two or more organ systems.	Patients who can benefit from more detailed observation or monitoring than can safely be provided on a general ward.
Patients with chronic impairment of one or more organ systems sufficient to restrict daily activities and who require support of an acute reversible failure of another organ system.	Patients no longer needing intensive care, but are not yet well enough to be returned to a general ward.
	Post-operative patients who need close monitoring for longer than a few hours.

Inappropriate admission

Apart from considerations of cost, inappropriate use of critical care facilities has other implications.[5] The patient may experience unnecessary suffering and loss of dignity. Relatives may also have to endure considerable emotional pressures. In some cases, treatment may simply prolong the process of dying or sustain life of doubtful quality, and in others the risks of interventions may far outweigh any potential benefits. To ensure a humane approach to the management of the critically ill and that limited resources are used appropriately, it is important to identify those patients who are most likely to benefit from intensive care and high dependency care, and to withhold or limit treatment when there is no prospect of recovery. It is also important to avoid admitting those who will make a good recovery without needless iatrogenic intervention.[6]

A patient's stated or written preference against intensive care should also be taken into account. Patients or their legal surrogates have the right to control what happens to them. Informed, rational and competent patients therefore have the right to refuse life-sustaining treatment. In addition, patients do not have the right to demand life-sustaining treatment when the clinician considers it inappropriate.[17]

As high mortality rates in the ICU and soon after discharge contribute significantly to the high costs of intensive care, this is a further reason why efforts to contain costs should concentrate on selecting patients with a reasonable chance of survival.[7] In practice, however, it is not usually acceptable to deny critically ill patients admission to intensive care, even when there is very little prospect of recovery from the acute illness:

- The long-term prognosis can be unpredictable and it is often difficult to make a precise diagnosis on initial assessment and the only appropriate course will be to admit the patient and assess the response after an appropriate period.

- A recent study comparing the costs of treating survivors with those for non-survivors estimated that the costs of treating non-survivors were approximately three times greater than those of survivors.[8]

- It is therefore important that the best use is made of intensive care resources and that, as far as possible, the most appropriate group of patients is admitted.

- Patients who can be expected to receive sustained benefit from intensive care in terms of quality and length of life should be admitted.

- All decisions should be made jointly by the patient/family, the intensive care team, and the referring team.

It was previously considered rational to deny admission to the critical care unit on the grounds of old age. Some elderly patients may have little or no chance of returning to an independent existence and there is evidence that age can affect long-term survival.[9] It appears, though, that physiological age is more important than chronological age in determining survival and that a careful assessment of the patient's pre-existing physiological reserve and co-morbidity, physical independence and social circumstances provides a better indication of the likely benefits of intensive care.[10] Limited physiological reserve is known to be an important determinant of mortality[11] and intensive care cannot replace lost reserve or reverse chronic ill health.

SUGGESTED ADMISSION CRITERIA FOR HDU AND ICU

Studies looking at the demand for HDUs have used various medical and surgical criteria for admission to the HDU and ICU.[12,13] The lists below represent the minimum criteria as used in some of these studies. The indications for admission may overlap with services provided by the renal unit, the thoracic HDU and the coronary care unit.

Medical criteria for admission to HDU

1. **Respiratory**

    (a) Patient requiring more than 40% oxygen on a fixed concentration mask.

    (b) Patient with an unstable respiratory condition likely to progress to a deterioration classified in (a) or uncontrolled respiratory failure.

    (c) Recently extubated patient (within last 6h). These patients would have been discharged from ICU.

    (d) Tracheostomy *in situ* requiring nursing attention more frequently than 2 hourly. These patients would have been discharged from ICU.

    (e) Intubated patients with no mechanical ventilatory support required throughout day or night.

    (f) Patient requiring the provision of continuous positive airway pressure (CPAP), intubated or unintubated.

    (g) Patient with minitracheostomy or similar device *in situ* requiring attention including physiotherapy at least 2 hourly.

2. **Cardiovascular**

    (a) Patient with a potentially unstable cardiovascular function requiring: (1) continuous ECG monitoring; (2) central venous pressure (CVP) monitoring; (3) an arterial line *in situ* for beat to beat pressure monitoring.

    (b) Patient with an unstable cardiovascular function or haemodynamic status due to haemorrhage – from whatever cause, including post-surgery gastrointestinal bleeding potentially uncontrolled by peripheral fluid replacement.

    (c) Patient with labile blood pressure (due to (b) or any intrinsic cause).

    (d) Patients requiring inotropic infusion.

3. **Renal**

    Patients at risk from developing renal failure, e.g. oliguria, in the post-operative period.

4. **Pain**

    Patients whose pain control could not be safely managed in the ward because of pre-existing disease.

Surgical criteria for admission to HDU

(a) Patient following surgery of an unexpected duration greater than 4 h.

(b) Patient following surgery incorporating unexpected blood loss greater than half the circulating blood volume.

Criteria for admission to ICU

(a) After surgery, patients requiring ventilation or who are haemodynamically unstable.

(b) Patients requiring mechanical ventilation from any cause.

(c) Treatment of metabolic encephalopathy.

(d) Patients requiring treatment of acute renal failure such as extracorporeal renal replacement therapy and who cannot be managed on the renal unit.

(e) Patients requiring resuscitation and optimisation before surgery.

Severity scoring indices, the best known of which is APACHE, are useful clinical tools in predicting probable outcome and in measuring the severity of a patient's condition. They are valuable for predicting the probability of outcome for a cohort of similar patients but not for an individual.[14] Kilpatrick et al.[15] studied admissions to a general ICU and found that 40% of patients were admitted with a predicted risk of mortality of less than 10% using the APACHE score. They suggest that patients with a low mortality risk might be better managed on an HDU. Although such scores will continue to be an important adjunct to clinical decision-making and frequently bear out the initial predicted outcome, they are insufficient as a basis for determining admission (or discharge). Indeed, most methods rely on data collected during the first 24 h of intensive care. In addition, there are inevitably some patients whose death or survival differs from the model's prediction and this invalidates their use as the only basis for deciding on admission (or refusal) for intensive care or high dependency care.

With regard to surgical patients, the selection of patients most likely to benefit from admission to the HDU varies between units and mainly follows local practice. Many of these patients are short stay but require careful observation in the immediate post-operative period. Admission criteria relate mainly to the risk of the operation being performed, the patient's age, the severity of the patient's illness, and the need for close post-operative observation. Obviously, patients of advanced age undergoing major surgery commonly pose this combination of circumstances. The risk scoring methods of APACHE II are reliable in the ICU but are not appropriate for HDU. POSSUM scores are a very useful indication of operative morbidity and mortality and may well be a better choice in the HDU.[16] However, it does not address the problem of assessment of surgical patients who do not require surgery.

The severity of critical illness and the high expense of providing critical care emphasise the importance of guidelines on admission and discharge. Appropriate admission guidelines are especially important given that there is some evidence and opinion to show that patients are admitted to intensive care by necessity in the absence of other, more appropriate, facilities such as high dependency care:[18]

- It would seem that medical and nursing opinion is still the most reasonable way to select patients for HDU care.

- The use of selection criteria for ICU admission has not developed sufficiently and is controversial.

- Admission criteria would not be identical between hospitals as many hospitals have different categories of patients requiring treatment.

- It is equally important to allow admission criteria to evolve to meet the needs of a changing patient population.

COMPREHENSIVE CRITICAL CARE

Management of surgical patients has become more complex now, as the patients are older and sicker. Developments in the field of surgery and anaesthetics have lead to more complex therapies and operations:

- These patients are more dependent on pre-operative optimization and post-operative care.

- At the same time there has been a reduction in the number of nursing staff in general wards due to recruitment problems.

- Added to this is the reduction of junior doctor working hours, which has lead to the shift system.

- There is loss of continuity of care, reduced working relationship between junior doctors and nurses.

All this leads to breakdown of communication that is vital in the care of the high risk patient.

Thus, we have patients with limited physiological reserve, who are vulnerable to sudden deterioration, which if not promptly treated can lead to catastrophy.

- Recent studies have shown that 40% of ICU admissions are potentially avoidable and about 55% of patients admitted to ICU had sub-optimal care prior to admission to the ICU.

- It was also shown that patients who were appropriately treated in the wards prior to ICU admission fared better.

- The difference in ICU mortality between the groups treated appropriately – 35% and those with sub-optimal care – 56%, is highly significant.[19]

- The 1993 NCEPOD report showed that two-thirds of peri-operative deaths occurred 3 or more days after surgery – in the ward, with cardio-pulmonary complications.

This highlights the principle 'prevention is better than cure'. Numerous studies have shown that there are premonitory signs and symptoms before the patients deteriorate catastrophically.[20] The aim should be to identify 'at risk' patients, establish appropriate monitoring and develop a system of 'red flag' to identify derangements of physiology so that there can be appropriate corrective measures.

In April 1999 the Department of Health established a review of adult critical care services. The expert group came up with the idea of 'comprehensive critical care', which is a new approach to patients based on the severity of illness. It recommends that the doors of intensive care should be opened up to export critical care skills beyond the ICUs to any area within the hospital where such skills are needed. This is the fundamental concept of critical care outreach. This outreach service has three main objectives:[21]

- to avert admission to ICU,

- to enable discharges from ICU,

- to share critical care skills with doctors and nurses in the wards.

The obvious first step, to avert admission to ICU, is for the ward staff looking after patients (at level 1 and 2 as discussed previously), to realise who is at risk of becoming critically ill. It is difficult to give an exhaustive list of patients who should be considered as 'at risk', but the following are commonly quoted by many outreach services as a good guide. They include:

- elderly patients,

- patients admitted as emergencies until stable,

- patients with pre-existing diseases,

- patients whose acute illness is particularly severe,

- patients who fail to progress after treatment,

- patient following ICU discharge,

- patients with decreased level of consciousness,

- patients needing massive blood transfusion.

THE EARLY WARNING SCORE FOR SURGICAL PATIENTS[22]

- The Early Warning Score was developed at the James Paget Hospital, Great Yarmouth, UK to aid the early recognition of patients at risk of becoming critically ill.

- It has been developed further at Queens Hospital, Burton-on-Trent resulting in the Modified Early Warning System (MEWS). Urine output was added to the early warning score to obtain the modified early warning score.

- Essentially the system is a tool, which enables ward-nursing staff to combine their routine observations to produce an aggregate physiological score.

- This dynamic scoring system is used to target appropriate help and treatments to the right patients at the right time.

- If the score remains persistently high then the critical care team may have to be involved.

Other similar 'physiological police' groups in various countries are: the medical emergency team; the patient at risk team and the critical care liaison service. The input from these teams may prevent an admission to the ICU and when admission becomes necessary it will be at an earlier stage of the patients illness.

Generally a MEWS score of > 3 is a trigger to call for senior help. Respiratory rate scores one or more in 97.5% of the observations in patients who have a total MEWS score > 4, making it the most sensitive indicator of a deteriorating patient. In comparison, temperature seems to be the least sensitive indicator, scoring > 0 in only 7% of the observations (table 16.1).

Table 16.1 – The modified early warning score (MEWS).

			Score			
3	**2**	**1**	**0**	**1**	**2**	**3**
Respiratory rate	< 8		9–14	15–20	21–29	> 30
Heart rate	< 40	40–50	51–100	101–110	111–129	> 130
Blood pressure (%) > 45	30	15	Normal for patient	15	30	> 45
Central nervous system			Alert	Responds to voice	Responds to pain	Unresponsive
Temperature	< 35.0		35–38.4		> 38.4	
Urine (ml/kg/h)	< 0.5	< 1		> 3		

ALERT

The other major aspect of the comprehensive critical care is to take the skills of the intensive care to the wards. To this effect the ALERT (acute life-threatening events – recognition and treatment) course is being implemented in many NHS hospitals. This course, run by a mutidisciplinary team led by intensivists is aimed at nurses in general wards and PRHOs. It is a 1-day course in acute care similar to the ACLS and ATLS, designed specifically to address the high level of sub-optimal ward care. It focuses on the anxieties of ward nurses and PRHOs and the areas of perceived weakness in the management of acutely ill patients and emphasizes on the recognition and early management of sick patients. It sets out a simple assessment and management system that is applicable to everyone.[23]

MEWS with the recently commissioned ALERT course should be able to identify at risk patients and provide a quantitative, objective and dynamic indication of the patient's status. Like the GCS the MEWS score can be used for better communication between staff. It also helps the nursing staff and junior doctors to pick up the sick patients at an early stage of their physiological derangement and implement appropriate therapy. This lead time (similar to the golden hour in acute trauma) in the management of patients should decrease the necessity of ICU/HDU admission of patients.

References

1. The Royal College of Anaesthetists. *National ITU Audit*. London: Royal College of Anaesthetists, 1992/1993.

2. Department of Health. *Comprehensive Critical Care. A Review of Adult Critical Care Services*. London: HMSO, 2000.

3. Crosby DL, Rees GAD. Provision of postoperative care in UK hospitals. *Ann R Coll Surg Engl* 1994; **76**: 14–18.

4. Franklin CM, Rackow EC, Mandami B *et al*. Decreases in mortality on a large urban medical service by facilitating access to critical care. *Arch Intern Med* 1988; **148**: 1403–5.

5. Jennett B. Inappropriate use of intensive care. *Br Med J* 1984; **289**: 1709–11.

6. Hinds CJ, Watson D. *Intensive Care. A Concise Textbook*, 2nd edn, 1996. London: Saunders.

7. Ridley S, Biggam M, Stone P. A cost-utility analysis of intensive therapy. *Anaesthesia* 1994; **49**: 192–6.

8. Atkinson A, Bihari D, Sithies M *et al*. Identification of futility in intensive care. *Lancet* 1994; **344**: 1203–6.

9. Ridley S, Jackson R, Findlay J, Wallace P. Long term survival after intensive care. *Br Med J* 1990; **301**: 1127–30.

10. Editorial: Intensive care for the elderly. *Lancet* 1991; **337**: 209–10.

11. Bion J. Rationing and triage in intensive care. In Vincent JL (ed.), *1995 Yearbook of Intensive Care and Emergency Medicine*. Springer Books.

12. Leeson-Payne CG, Aitkenhead AR. A prospective study to assess the demand for a high dependency unit. *Anaesthesia* 1995; **50**: 383–7.

13. Ryan DW, Bayly PJM, Weldon OGW, Jingree M. A prospective two-month audit of the lack of provision of a high-dependency unit and its impact on intensive care. *Anaesthesia* 1997; **52**: 265–75.

14. Teres D, Lemeshow S. Why severity models should be used with caution. *Crit Care Med* 1994; **10**: 93–110.

15. Kilpatrick A, Ridley S, Plenderleith L. A changing role for intensive therapy: is there a case for high dependency care? *Anaesthesia* 1994; **49**: 666–70.

16. Jones DR, Copeland GP, de Cossart L. Comparison of POSSUM and APACHE II for prediction of outcome from a surgical high dependency unit. *Br J Surg* 1992; **79**: 1293–6.

17. Ruark JE, Raffin TA. Initiating and withdrawing life support: principles and practice in adult medicine. *N Engl J Med* 1988; **318**: 25–30.

18. Metcalfe A, McPherson K. *Study of Intensive Care in England 1993*, 1995. London: HMSO.

19. McQuillan P, Pilkington S, Allan A *et al*. Confidential inquiry into quality of care before admission to intensive care. *Br Med J* 1998; **316**: 1853–8.

20. Franklin C, Matthew J. Developing strategies to prevent in hospital cardiac arrest: analyzing responses of physicians and nurses in the hours before the event. *Crit Care Med* 1994; **22**: 244–7.

21. Department of Health. *Comprehensive Critical Care – Review of Adult Critical Care Services*, 1997.

22. Stenhouse CW, Bion JF. Outreach: a hospital–wide approach to critical illness. *Yearbook of Intensive Care and Emergency Medicine*, 2001: 661–75.

23. Smith G. ALERT Course Manual, 1st edn, October 2000.

17

THE MEANING OF RISK

- Risk is usually defined as a hazard of loss, or alternatively as the probability of incurring a bad consequence, or misfortune. It is implicitly negative and is suggestive of a potential danger or hazard and thus is associated with loss and not gain.

- In 1983 the Royal Society defined *risk* as 'the probability that a particular event occurs during a stated period of time or results from a particular challenge'. They defined a *hazard* as a situation that could lead to harm. The chance or likelihood of this occurring is its associated *risk*.[1]

- It is widely recognised that individuals tend to evaluate risks, not solely on statistical data but on many other subjective qualitative aspects of risks. It is also evident that the assessment and perception of risk is subconscious, subjective, personality dependant and fails to follow any rational or methodical pattern.[2]

IDENTIFYING RISKS

- Identification of the common potential hazards is not usually a problem but it may be difficult to recognise rare complications particularly with newly introduced drugs or if there is long lead-time between a treatment and a complication.

- The timing of any adverse outcomes can have significant effect on the way a particular risk is perceived. Early complications, for example, often have a greater impact than those that are delayed which tend to have a diminished perceived risk value.

- The duration of any adverse outcome can also affect risk perception. Something that is transient like post-operative pain will obviously have less impact than something more permanent in nature like death or disability. Furthermore, those complications that are easily treated tend to have downgraded perceived risk severity values.

PERCEIVING RISK

Many previous studies on risk perception have attempted to characterise those aspects thought relevant to the way we evaluate risk. The main criteria of risks that consciously and subconsciously contribute to the way risks are perceived include:

- magnitude,
- severity,
- vulnerability,
- controllability,
- familiarity,
- acceptability,
- framing effect.

Risk probability or magnitude

- The current accepted method of expressing risk probability or magnitude of an adverse outcome is in terms of the mathematical probability of an adverse event occurring.

- Estimates of clinical probabilities are usually based on their frequency of occurrence in previously published studies. Risk probabilities quoted need to be interpreted with caution as accuracy requires large sample sizes, and patient populations studied in other countries may not be applicable to our own.

- No matter what the actual probability value is, various factors can influence how large, significant or inevitable a risk is perceived to be.

Distortion of the magnitude of risk can be due to two different types of error known as availability and compression bias.

Availability bias (also known as exposure or publication bias) is an overestimation of risk to over exposure or publicity of usually rare, catastrophic or dramatic events. Probabilities of events are up or downgraded according to the ease with which instances of similar events can be recalled:

- Thus rare events are more likely to be sensationalised and are therefore perceived to be more common than they actually are and conversely, common events are less dramatic, less sensational and therefore underestimated.

Information availability on a hazard can affect risk perception: for example, widespread media coverage of airline crashes increases public anxiety about the risks of airline transport when compared to car travel which is vastly more dangerous in terms of fatalities per kilometre travelled.

Compression bias occurs because of the vast ranges that probabilities can span; patients overestimate small risks and underestimate large ones. It is difficult to communicate and comprehend rare risks:

- Thus people underestimate the risk of mortality in travelling by bicycle and overestimate the mortality risk of train travel.

Risk severity

This is subjective and perception dependant. The worst outcomes are death or disability and these obviously have the greatest impact on risk perception.

One mathematical concept used in the past as an attempt to analyse processes involved in risk perception, was to compare different risks using expectation value, which is calculated as the product of probability and severity:[3]

$$\text{Expectation value} = \text{probability} \times \text{severity}.$$

This is obviously only of use if one can assign a numerical value to severity.

However, it is a considerable oversimplification of the issues we consider when evaluating a risk for ourselves:

- For example, risks with a very low probability but high severity, for example death or disability, are perceived worse than risks with a higher probability and less severe outcome that have the same expectation value.

Furthermore, it can be very difficult to assign realistic representative numerical values for severity of outcomes that are subjective and perceiver dependant.

Vulnerability

Vulnerability is the extent to which people believe an event could happen to them or alternatively is the degree of immunity one possesses to a risk. Generally we tend to exhibit unrealistic optimism and a feeling of immunity or invincibility so people tend not to behave cautiously. Feeling invulnerable, we underestimate or downgrade our own risk but overestimate the risk to others:

- For example, one might fear more the catastrophic but rare risk of nuclear accident than the common but minor risk of passive smoking.

Controllability

The possibility of something adverse happening that cannot be controlled magnifies the perceived severity of the risk; we like to be in control; if we can exert some element of control then we feel we can exert influence and minimise the chance or even prevent the event from occurring. The perception of being in control or having choice downgrades the perceived severity of the risk:[4]

- For example, major risks may be faced regularly (for example, with smoking or hang-gliding) particularly if individuals deem themselves invulnerable risk-takers and perceive that they are in control of the risks which they could avoid if they so wished.

- For example, we are often faced with the necessity of travelling from A to B with certain time constraints forcing the use of a particular mode of public transport offering no other options. Be it flying, rail travel, or the motorcar most of us accept the risks associated partly through necessity and partly through the perception of being in control and exerting some kind of choice.

We are much more willing to accept higher risk levels if they are undertaken voluntarily than if they are imposed.

On the other hand, involuntary or imposed risks are significantly less acceptable or tolerable:

- For example, risks from passive smoking, or air pollution; the lack of control incites resentment.

Familiarity

Familiarity of exposure and overconfidence of the extent and accuracy of our knowledge desensitises us to risks, whereas unfamiliar risks incite a greater degree of fear or dread. This distortion is defined in risk terminology as miscalibration bias.

Acceptability or dread

Individual attitudes, upbringing, economic situations, and cultural setting, significantly affect this concept of fear or dread:

- The loss of a lower limb, for example, might impose greater fear in a professional footballer than an office worker.

- More graphically being eaten alive by great white shark usually embodies far greater dread than being killed by road traffic accident, even though the final outcome is the same.

The more different characteristics there are embodied in a hazard, the more likely individuals' risk assessments will differ. However likely, severe, controllable, or familiar, acceptable the risk seems and however vulnerable or immune the individual feels will all depend upon a variety of personal experiences and upon the cultural context within which the perceiver operates.

Framing effect or framing bias

This is how differences in the presentation of risk information can affect perception.

Simply providing risk information on its own is insufficient to change behaviour, but factual information presented effectively can help achieve this:

- In other words, it not what is presented but how risk is presented that can have the greatest effect on risk perception and thereby influence behaviour.

It is well recognised that differences in the presentation of risk information can strongly affect the perception of risk in both lay people and doctors and thereby influence decision making.[5] The order in which one chooses to discuss the advantages or disadvantages of an intervention may have an impact on a patients perception and final decision and may be one of the many ways in which clinicians can sway patients final decision on the acceptability of treatments:

- For example, emphasising positive aspects before discussing the risks may be more likely to persuade an individual to accept a particular therapy.

- Furthermore, adding emphasis to the positive aspects results in a greater uptake; a therapy reported to be 60% effective would be evaluated more favourably than by reporting a 40% failure rate, even though the two statements are objectively equal.

- Similarly a treatment with 10% mortality will be better received if phrased as having 90% chance of survival. This is known as positive framing.[5]

COMMUNICATING RISK LEVELS

At present there is no universal accepted method for the presentation of probability information in a format that is readily understood. We have yet to find a format that conveys population risk data into clinical risk information that is readily understandable by the individual.[6]

Because the range of probabilities when expressing risk can be extremely large, and because risk probability data is often only accurate to within an order of magnitude, integer logarithmic scales are often used as a way of presenting risk magnitude information in a more manageable format.

A number of different integer logarithm based risk scales have been suggested by various authors in verbal, numerical and graphical formats:

- Examples of logarithmic scales in everyday use include the Richter scale for earthquake magnitude, the pH scale for hydrogen ion concentration and the decibel scale for sound intensity.

Table 17.1 – Easily understood risk scales.

Risk level 1 in ...	Calmans verbal scale	Calmans descriptive terms	Community cluster 1 person in a ...
1–9			
10–99	High	Frequent, significant	Family
100–999	Moderate		Street
1000–9 999	Low	Tolerable, reasonable	Village
10 000–99 999	Very low		Small town
100 000–999 999	Minimal	Acceptable	Large town
1 000 000–9 999 999	Negligible	Insignificant safe	City

- All the numerical scales are extremely limited in their use for conveying risk magnitude particularly to the layperson; big numbers are simply being substituted for smaller numbers with a similar lack of meaning.

- On the other hand Calmans verbal scale[2] and his descriptive terms, or the community cluster classification[7] are much more useful because of their validity and relevance to the layperson. This is illustrated in table 17.1.

- Others have suggested using the National Lottery and the probabilities of the various winning ball combinations as a scale of risk that might be more understandable to the lay person:[8]

    1 in 57 = 3 balls,   1 in 55 491 = 5 balls,   1 in 13 983 816 = 6 balls,

    1 in 1032 = 4 balls,   1 in 2 330 636 = 5 balls + bonus.

WHAT IS HIGH RISK?

Graphical risk ladders have even more impact and meaning when individual examples of clinical risks are displayed alongside examples of every day risks that are readily accepted on a daily basis[9] (figure 17.1):

- Recently the 1 : 100 000 risk level was deemed minimal or even *acceptable*[7] and suggested a risk level of less than 1 : 1 000 000 as being 'safe'.

- Examples of risks below this '*acceptable*' frequency of 1 : 100 000 include the risk of death by murder in 1 year at 1 : 100 000 and the risk of death by railway accident at 1 : 500 000.

It is enlightening that many of us unwittingly accept the risk of death by road traffic accident in 1 year at 1 in 8000[10] on our daily journeys to and from work.

- This level of risk below 1 in 1000 is deemed '*tolerable or reasonable*'.[2]

Some workers however, strongly believe that there is no single level of risk that is universally acceptable.[4] For example, some individuals will choose what they

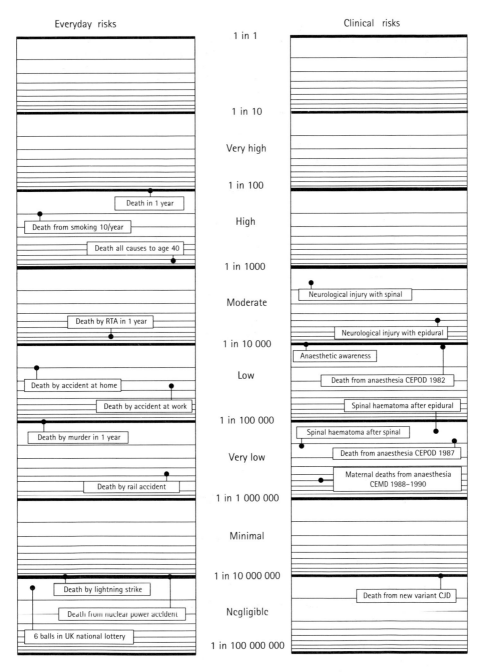

Everyday risks

Clinical risks

1 in 1

1 in 10

Very high

1 in 100

Death in 1 year

High

Death from smoking 10/year

Death all causes to age 40

1 in 1000

Neurological injury with spinal

Moderate

Death by RTA in 1 year

Neurological injury with epidural

1 in 10 000

Anaesthetic awareness

Low

Death from anaesthesia CEPOD 1982

Death by accident at home

Death by accident at work

Spinal haematoma after epidural

1 in 100 000

Spinal haematoma after spinal

Death by murder in 1 year

Death from anaesthesia CEPOD 1987

Very low

Maternal deaths from anaesthesia
CEMD 1988–1990

Death by rail accident

1 in 1 000 000

Minimal

1 in 10 000 000

Death by lightning strike

Death from new variant CJD

Death from nuclear power accident

Negligible

6 balls in UK national lottery

1 in 100 000 000

Figure 17.1 – Risk ladder relating anaesthetic risks to everyday risks (reproduced with permission from Ref. 10).

perceive to be the best alternative for them, and the risk associated with that choice must therefore be acceptable to them. In other words, risk magnitude can often have secondary importance to other subjective criteria involved in the perception of risk.

RISK–BENEFIT ANALYSIS

Risk benefit analysis involves a full assessment of risks and comparing and balancing this with the potential gain.

It is a perception dependant process that is particularly reliant on an individual's analysis of those advantages and disadvantages of accepting a particular hazard for the chance of a particular gain.

The mnemonic **BRAN** offers a useful approach when assessing the risks of a course of action and includes the **B**enefits, **R**isks, **A**lternatives, and what would happen if you did **N**othing!

What are the Benefits?

- Identify the benefits.

- Assess the likelihood of benefit.

- Assess the perceived value of the benefit.

- How soon could benefit occur.

- Is the benefit permanent or temporary.

What are the Risks?

- Identify the risks.

- Assess the likelihood or probability of risk.

- Assess the perceived value of the risk.

- How soon could the risk occur.

- Is the risk permanent or temporary.

What are the Alternatives?

What if you do Nothing?

The **BRAN** approach may be useful in anaesthetic practice. However, one must know what the risks are before this can be applied to discussions with and management of individual patients.

In the year 2000, the risk of dying in the first 28 days following emergency and non–emergency surgery in the UK was 1 in 25 and 1 in 200, respectively.[11]

Table 17.2 – Examples of the risks of surgery in the UK.

Statistic	Incidence (%)	Risk
30-day mortality following cardio-oesophagectomy	10	1 in 10
30-day mortality following fractured neck of femur	9.07	1 in 11
30-day perioperative mortality – emergency surgery	3.87	1 in 25
30-day perioperative mortality – non-emergency surgery	0.48	1 in 200

Transposing these figures to the risk ladder in figure 17.1 shows that the risks of undergoing a surgical procedure are not insignificant (table 17.2).

Patient's (and indeed clinical staff's) perception of risk is influenced by many factors and understanding of probabilities and percentage chances of significant complications is poor.

References

1. Royal Society. *Risk Assessment: Report of a Royal Society Working Party*, 1983. Royal Society, London.

2. Calman KC. Cancer: science and society and the communication of risk. *Br Med J* 1996; **313**: 799–802.

3. Broadbent DE. Psychology of risk. In Cooper MG (ed.) *Risk: Man-made Hazards to Man*. Oxford: Clarendon Press, 1985.

4. Keeney RL. Understanding life-threatening risks. *Risk Anal* 1995; **15**: 627–37.

5. Malenka DJ, Baron JA, Johansen S *et al*. The framing effect of relative and absolute risk. *J Gen Intern Med* 1993; **8**: 543–8.

6. Edwards A, Prior L. Communication about risk – dilemmas for general practitioners. *Br J Gen Prac* 1997; **47**: 739–42.

7. Calman KC, Royston HD. Risk language and dialects. *Br Med J* 1997; **315**: 939–42.

8. Barclay P, Costigan S, Davies M. Lottery can be used to show risk (letter). *Br Med J* 1998; **316**: 124.

9. Adams AM, Smith AF. Risk perception and communication: recent developments and implications for anaesthesia. *Anaesthesia* 2001; **56**: 745–55.

10. *BMA Guide to Living with Risk*. Harmondsworth: Penguin, 1990.

11. http://www.doh.gov.uk/nhsperformanceindicators.

INDEX

ABC system, resuscitation 89
abdomen
    abscesses 175
    compartment syndrome 183–184
    pain 59–60
    sepsis 173
    surgery
        gastrointestinal 165–178
        respiratory risk 32 (Table)
ABO incompatible blood transfusions,
        mortality 220
abscesses, percutaneous drainage 175
acceptability
    risk levels 244
    treatments 243
accident and emergency departments,
        patients from 77
acidosis 96–97
    aortic aneurysm surgery 160
activated neutrophils, reperfusion injury
        prevention 162
acute pain services (APS) 51–52
    techniques 56–57
acute renal failure 179–195
    renal support 192–194
acute tubular necrosis 180
Adamkiewicz, artery of 158
adenosine, stress testing 21
admission, analgesia 56
admission criteria, HDU and ICU 227–237
adrenaline
    hypertrophic cardiomyopathy 207

local anaesthesia 70, 72–73
    peri-operative optimisation 122
adrenaline (endogenous), ageing 106
adrenal suppression, etomidate 84
adult respiratory distress syndrome, ketamine
        88
aeroplane crashes, availability bias in risk
        perception 240–241
afterload
    aortic regurgitation 145
    mitral stenosis 147
afterload mismatch, aortic stenosis 143
ageing 101–106
    by aortic aneurysm surgery 154
    see also elderly patients
airflow obstruction, value of testing 34
airways
    aspiration prevention 168
    elderly patients 103–104, 112
    management 82–83
    manipulation and haemodynamics
        136
    patient transfer 78
albumin, ageing 107
aldosterone, ageing 105
ALERT course 236
algorithm controlled opioids 57
ambulatory electrocardiographic monitoring
        18–19, 24, 203
American College of Cardiologists,
        ACC/AHA guidelines, pre-operative
        assessment 13–15

American College of Physicians, pulmonary function testing 36
American Heart Association, ACC/AHA guidelines, pulmonary function testing 13–15
American Society of Anesthesiologists
　ASA status classification 9–10, 30, 46
　task force on blood transfusions 222
aminoglycosides, renal failure 184
anaemia 215–255
anaesthetic agents 83–88
　see also inhalational anaesthetic agents; local anaesthetic agents; specific drugs
anaesthetic rooms 89
anaesthetists, competence and clinical risk 2
analgesia 51–63
　elderly patients, post-operative 113–114
　thoracic surgery 60
anastomoses, gastrointestinal surgery 169–170, 176
anatomical site of surgery
　analgesia 58–61
　respiratory complications and risk 32–33, 173
　　pain 53
aneurysms, aorta 153–154
angiography
　coronary 24–25, 130, 203
　mitral regurgitation 147
angioplasty, coronary 24, 25, 131, 205
angiotensin converting enzyme, clinical risk and 3
angiotensin converting enzyme inhibitors 132
　renal failure 184
angiotensin receptor antagonists 132
animal studies
　ketamine 87, 88
　thiopentone 87
antacids 168
anterior resection, bowel anastomoses 169
antibiotics, renal failure 184
anticoagulants
　epidural anaesthesia and 54, 61
　prosthetic heart valves 208–209
　regional anaesthesia 66–68
antihypertensive drugs 6, 206

antitachycardia devices 210–211
aorta, surgery
　emergency operations 17, 153–164
　Goldman's Cardiac Risk Index 10
　pulmonary artery catheters 91
　see also cross-clamping
aortic regurgitation 8, 141, 144–146, 208
aortic stenosis 141, 142–144, 208
　clinical risk 7–8
　epidural anaesthesia 60, 144
APACHE scoring systems 13, 232
aprotinin, renal failure 184
APSs see acute pain services
arbitrator/coordinators, emergencies 43
arbutamine, stress testing 20–21
arginine, immune system stimulation 172
arrhythmias 209–211
　adrenaline 73
　clinical risk and 8
　local anaesthetic agents 69
　valvular heart disease 142
arterial blood gas analysis
　aortic aneurysm surgery 159
　pre-operative 37
　　aortic aneurysm surgery 155
arterial lines 90
　aortic aneurysm surgery 156
arterial oxygen content, anaemia 215
arteries
　of Adamkiewicz 158
　ageing 102
arteriovenous fistulae, regional anaesthesia 73–74
artificial heart valves 208–209
ASA status classification (American Society of Anesthesiologists) 9–10, 30, 46
aspiration risk, gastrointestinal surgery 167–168
aspirin
　platelet function 67
　pre-operative 131–132
　regional anaesthesia 67, 112
asthma
　clinical risk 32
　coronary vasodilators 21
atherosclerosis 108
　cardiac risk 4

atracurium, respiratory risk 33
atrial fibrillation, mitral stenosis 147
atrial natriuretic factor 192
    ageing 105
atropine, dobutamine stress echocardiography
    22
audit, NCEPOD on 47–48
Austin Flint murmur 145
Australian Working Party group (NHMRC),
    epidural anaesthesia 54
autologous blood transfusions 219
    aortic aneurysm surgery 161
autonomic ganglia, local anaesthetic agents
    69
autopsy *see* post-mortem review
availability bias, risk assessment 240–241

bacterial endocarditis prophylaxis 209
bacterial infections, blood transfusion risk
    218
bactericidal permeability increasing protein
    218
balanced analgesia *see* multi-modal analgesia
balloon pumps, intra-aortic 133, 211
balloons *see* pulmonary capillary wedge
    pressure
balloon valvuloplasty 208
basal metabolic rate, ageing 106
benefits *vs* risks 246–247
β₂-adrenoceptors
    ageing 102, 105, 106
    dopexamine 122
β-adrenergic blockers
    emergency surgery 206
    hypertension 7
    intra-operative myocardial ischaemia 137
    pre-operative 131, 132, 205
biases, risk perception 240–243
bicarbonate, rhabdomyolysis 187
blood flow
    cerebral, ageing 106
    coronary arteries 134
        anaemia 217
    kidney *see* renal blood flow
blood gases *see* arterial blood gas analysis
blood loss
    epidural anaesthesia 72

hypothermia 81
    transfusion for 93–94
    see also haemorrhage
blood pressure
    warning of deterioration 235 (Table)
    see also hypertension; hypotension
blood (product) transfusions 93–94, 217–223
    aortic aneurysm surgery 159, 161
    confounding fluid therapy studies 91–92
    gastrointestinal surgery 170–171
    haemolytic reactions 219–220
    NCEPOD recommendations for 43
bone marrow depression 216
bowel cancer surgery, surgeons as risk factor
    1–2
bowel obstruction 175
    aspiration risk 167
    nitrous oxide 168
brachial plexus block 59
    for arteriovenous fistula 73
bradycardia, 'paradoxical' 95
BRAN approach, risk-benefit analysis
    246–247
bronchospasm
    coronary vasodilators 21
    prediction by pulmonary function testing
        34
    surgical risk 32
bupivacaine, epidural anaesthesia 57
    patient-controlled 58

calcium channel blockers 192
    pre-operative 131, 132
Calmans verbal and descriptive scales, risk
    communication 244
cancer recurrence, blood transfusions
    170–171, 219
capacity limited drugs, ageing 107
capillaries, anaemia 216
cardiac arrest, acute renal failure after 182
cardiac enzyme measurement 211
cardiac glycosides, digitalis 206
cardiac index
    peri-operative optimisation 120, 122
    peri-operative risk 118
cardiac output
    ageing 102

cardiac output (*contd*)
  anaemia 216
  aortic aneurysm surgery 160
  dopamine 191
  peri-operative risk 118
  renal failure 185
cardiac risk 4–25, 129, 199–200
cardiac surgery
  haemofiltration trial 193
  renal failure 182–183
cardiogenic shock 94
cardiology 199–214
  see also heart
cardiomyopathy 207
  epidural anaesthesia 60
cardio-oesophagectomy, risk 247 (Table)
cardiopulmonary bypass, renal function 187
cardiopulmonary reserve, cardiac risk 4
carotid endarterectomy, local anaesthesia 73
cell savers, blood transfusions 161
central nervous system
  ageing 105–106
  dialysis 193
  local anaesthetic agents 68–69
  thiopentone 83–84
  see also neurological injury; neurosurgery
central venous catheters 90
  aortic aneurysm surgery 156
  valvular heart disease 142
central venous pressure 90
cerebral blood flow, ageing 106
Chagas disease, transfusion risk 218
Charing Cross protocol, renal failure
  prevention 189
children, NCEPOD recommendations for
  43
chloride, metabolic acidosis 97
chronic obstructive pulmonary disease
  blood transfusions and 221
  clinical risk 32
Clinical Negligence Scheme for Trusts, on
  training 45
clinical volume, *vs* risk 1–2
clinician-based patient assessment, clinical
  risk 17–18
clonidine 56, 70–71
closing volume (lungs), ageing 103

coagulation defects
  aortic aneurysm surgery 159, 161
  hypothermia 81, 82
  regional anaesthesia 66–68
  see also anticoagulants
cocaine 69
colloids 91–92
  aortic aneurysm surgery 155
  renal failure 184–185
colon, perforation 176
colorectal surgery
  Possum score performance 13
  surgeons as risk factor 1–2
communication
  decisions to operate 46
  failure 234
  NCEPOD on 44–45
  of risk levels 243–244
community-acquired acute renal failure 182
community cluster classification, risk
  communication 244
compartment syndrome, abdomen 183–184
compliance (lungs), ageing 103
comprehensive critical care 234
compression bias, risk perception 241
computed tomography, NCEPOD
  recommendations for 43
computerised ST segment monitoring 137,
  211
conduction defects 209–211
  ageing 102
congenital heart disease 209
consciousness, level of, warning of
  deterioration 235 (Table)
consent
  elderly patients 112
  post-mortem examinations 48
  see also patient refusal
consultants
  NCEPOD on 43–44
  see also senior help requests
consultation, NCEPOD on 44
continuous venovenous haemofiltration
  192–194
contrast media
  acute renal failure 182, 184, 187, 188
  dopamine and 191

controllability, risk perception 241
coordinators (arbitrator/coordinators),
    emergencies 43
coronary angiography 24–25, 130,
    203
coronary angioplasty 24, 25, 131, 205
coronary arteries
    ageing 102–103
    blood flow 134
      anaemia 217
    occlusion 127–128
      see also myocardial infarction
    surgery, anaesthetists' competence and
      clinical risk 2
coronary artery bypass grafting 24, 25
    blood transfusions, morbidity 220
    pre-operative 130–131
    pulmonary artery catheters and 91
coronary artery disease 127–140
    clinical risk 5–6
      predictors 15, 128–129, 200
    elderly patients 110
    epidural anaesthesia 54, 137
coronary perfusion pressure 134
coronary revascularisation
    non-invasive testing and 6
    pre-operative 130–131, 204
    recent history of 201, 204
    see also coronary angioplasty; coronary
      artery bypass grafting
coronary vascular resistance 134
coronary vasodilators, stress testing 21
costs
    blood transfusions 219
    critical care 230
cough, pain on 53
creatinine clearance
    acute renal failure 180, 181
    ageing 104
    dialysis 193
cricoid pressure 168
critical care
    comprehensive 234
    outreach 234
    pre-operative, NCEPOD on 46–47
    see also high dependency units; intensive
      care units

cross-clamping of aorta 158–160
    renal function 187
    unclamping 159–160
crystalloids 91–92
    aortic aneurysm surgery 155
    renal failure 184–185
cytokines, blood transfusions 218–219

decisions to operate 46
defibrillators, implanted 210–211
dehydration, elderly patients 110
Department of Health, levels of care
    227–228
desflurane 86
dextran
    haematoma risk in epidural anaesthesia 68
    renal failure 184
diabetes mellitus, clinical risk and 8
dialysis
    intermittent 192–193
    see also arteriovenous fistulae
diamorphine
    epidural anaesthesia 57
      patient-controlled 58
    intravenous 56
digitalis 206
2,3-diphosphoglycerate
    anaemia 216
    stored blood 217
dipyridamole, stress testing 21, 23, 24, 202
diuretics, on kidney 184, 187–188, 190
dobutamine
    aortic aneurysm surgery 160
    aortic regurgitation 145–146
    mitral regurgitation 149
    pulmonary hypertension 150
    resuscitation 94
    stress testing 20–21
      echocardiography 21–22, 24, 202
dopamine
    aortic aneurysm surgery 160
    renal protection 190–191
dopexamine 122
    aortic aneurysm surgery 160
    on kidney 188–189
    peri-operative optimisation 121, 122
duration of surgery, respiratory risk 33

Early Warning Score, critical illness 235
echocardiography
    dobutamine stress testing 21–22, 24,
        202
    left ventricular ejection fraction 23
    mitral regurgitation 147–148
    NCEPOD on availability 47
    see also transoesophageal echocardiography
ejection fraction
    left ventricle 23
    mitral regurgitation 148
elastance, lungs, ageing 103
elderly patients 101–116
    adrenaline 70
    cardiac risk 5
    critical care 230
    fluid therapy 46, 93, 113
    general anaesthesia 111–113
    mortality 42
    NCEPOD recommendations for 43, 46
    regional anaesthesia 74, 111, 112
    renal failure 108, 183
    respiratory risk 31
    statistics 109
elective admission, elective surgery,
        NCEPOD definitions 48
electrocardiography
    ambulatory monitoring 18–19, 24, 203
    exercise stress testing 20, 23–24, 130
    peri-operative 211
electrocautery, pacemakers 210
electrolytes, urine, acute renal failure 180
emergencies 77–78
    admission, NCEPOD definition 48
    analgesia 56
    antihypertensive drugs 206
    cardiac risk management 201
    coordinators 43
    coronary artery disease 133
    fluid therapy, NCEPOD on 46
    mortality of surgery 247 (Table)
    operations on aorta 17, 153–164
    staff availability 45
emergency surgery
    'ASA' status classification 10
    NCEPOD definition 48
    risk of 17

emergency theatres, NCEPOD
        recommendations 43
emphysema, pulmonary function testing
        36
endocarditis prophylaxis 209
endometrial cancer, North American
        Negroes 3
endothelin antagonists 192
enflurane 85, 86
enteral nutrition 172
Entonox 56, 62
enzyme measurement, cardiac enzymes 211
epidural anaesthesia 51, 54, 57–58
    aortic stenosis 60, 144
    benefits 71–72
    complications 61, 66, 73
    coronary artery disease 54, 137
    elderly patients 112–113
        post-operative care 113–114
    gastrointestinal surgery 169
    opioids 57, 60, 70
    patient-controlled, incident pain 61–62
    on respiratory complications 173
    risk levels 245 (Fig.)
    on stress response to surgery 174–175
    thorax 60
epinephrine *see* adrenaline
erythropoietin
    response 216
    therapy 222
esmolol, intra-operative myocardial ischaemia
        137
ethics, critical care admission 229–230
ethnicity, on clinical risk 3
etomidate 84
exercise stress testing 20, 23–24, 130,
        201–202
exercise tolerance 15–16
    exercise stress testing 20
    respiratory risk 31
expectation value 241
expiratory reserve volume, ageing 103
exposure bias, risk assessment 240–241

familiarity, risk perception 242
fear, risk perception 242
felypressin 70

femoral neck fracture
    mortality of surgery 247 (Table)
    peri-operative optimisation 120
    volume loading 92
fentanyl 85
    epidural anaesthesia 57, 70
'fitness for surgery' 25
    pulmonary function testing for 35
flow limited drugs, ageing 107
fluid balance
    aged kidney 104–105
    elderly patients 110
        post-operative 113
fluid therapy 91–94
    aortic aneurysm surgery 155
    elderly patients
        intra-operative 93
        post-operative 113
        pre-operative 46
    gastrointestinal surgery 170
    metabolic acidosis from 97
    pre-operative, NCEPOD on 46
    renal failure 187
    resuscitation 89
forced expiratory volume '1'
    predicted post-operative 36
    pre-operative 34, 35
forced vital capacity, pre-operative 35
fractures
    femoral neck *see* femoral neck fracture
    metabolic activity of 96
framing effect, risk perception 243
free fractions of drugs, ageing 107
frusemide
    Charing Cross protocol 189
    on kidney 187–188
functional capacity *see* exercise tolerance
functional residual capacity
    ageing 103
    pain on 52–53

gastrointestinal surgery 165–178
gender
    cardiac risk 5
    clinical risk 2–3
genetics, on clinical risk 3
gentamicin, renal failure 184

glomerular atrophy, ageing 104
glomerular filtration rate, renal failure 181
glutamine supplements 172
glycosides, digitalis 206
Goldman's Cardiac Risk Index 10–11, 30
graduated patient care 229
guidelines provision, NCEPOD on 44

haematocrit
    coronary artery bypass grafting, morbidity
        220
    oxygen delivery 215
haematoma
    epidural 67
    spinal, risk levels 245 (Fig.)
haemodialysis, arteriovenous fistulae, regional
        anaesthesia 73–74
haemodynamics
    acute anaemia 216
    ageing 106
    aorta cross-clamping 158–159
    coronary arteries 134
    high dependency unit admission criteria
        231
    peri-operative 119–120
haemofiltration 192–194, 195
haemoglobin
    arterial oxygen content 215
    levels for transfusion 220–221, 222–223
haemolytic reactions, blood transfusions
        219–220
haemorrhage 77
    anaesthesia and 89
    congenital heart disease 209
    high dependency unit admission criteria
        231
    see also blood loss
haemorrhagic shock, traumatic shock *vs* 95–96
halothane 85–86
hazards, defined 239
head injuries 88
heart 199–214
    ageing 101–103, 108
    anaemia 216, 217
    clinical risk 4–25, 118
        respiratory risk 30–31
    epidural anaesthesia 60, 71

heart (*contd*)
    high dependency unit admission criteria 231
    hypothermia 81
    inhalational agents on 86
    ketamine 84, 87
    local anaesthesia 72–73
        agents 69
    see also cardiac surgery
heart failure
    clinical risk and 7
    peri-operative management 206–207
heart rate
    pulmonary hypertension 150
    warning of deterioration 235 (Table)
help requests (addressed to seniors) 44, 46
heparin
    epidural anaesthesia and 61, 67–68
    prosthetic heart valves 208–209
hepatic clearance of drugs, ageing 107
hepatitis B, hepatitis C, blood transfusion risks 218
hepatocellular function, ageing 105
high dependency units
    admission criteria 227–237
    advantages 228–229
    elderly patients 114
    vs intensive care units 229
    NCEPOD recommendations 43
    patients from 77
    Possum score performance 13
high volume haemofiltration 194, 195
hip *see* femoral neck fracture
histamine receptor antagonists 168
HIV infection, blood transfusion risk 218
homologous blood transfusions, aortic aneurysm surgery 161
hormones, ageing 106
hospital-acquired acute renal failure 182
hospitals, facilities required 42–43
Huffners constant 215
human immunodeficiency virus infection, blood transfusion risk 218
hypercapnia, clinical risk 37
hyperoncotic acute renal failure 184
hypertension
    cardiac risk 6–7

epidural anaesthesia 71
haemodynamics 135
pre-operative management 205–206
hypertrophic cardiomyopathy 207
    epidural anaesthesia 60
hyperventilation, raised intracranial pressure 88
hypokalaemia, heart failure 206
hypotension
    acute renal failure 182
    aorta cross-clamp release 160
    elderly patients 111
    epidural anaesthesia 58, 61, 66
    hypertension patients 205
    propofol 84
hypothermia 80–82, 111
    gastrointestinal surgery 167
    see also warming
hypovolaemia
    gastrointestinal surgery 170
    heart failure 206
    hypertrophic cardiomyopathy 207
    see also shock
hypoxia
    elderly patients 112
    general anaesthesia 86
    pain on 53
    peri-operative 118
    shock 96
hypoxic reperfusion 162

iatrogenic acute renal failure 182
ileus, epidural anaesthesia 72, 169
immune system
    dopamine on 191
    nutritional stimulation 172
immunosuppression, blood transfusions 218–219
impedance *vs* resistance, pulmonary vasculature 150
implanted defibrillators 210–211
incentive spirometry 174
incident pain 53, 61–62
incisions *see* anatomical site of surgery
induction of anaesthesia
    agents 83–84
    elderly patients 107–108, 112
    gastrointestinal surgery 168

infections
  blood transfusions
    from immunosuppression 219
    transmission 218
  epidural anaesthesia, reduction 72
  gender on clinical risk 2
inflammatory bowel disease 175
inflammatory response, blood transfusions
    218–219
infusions
  dopamine 190
  frusemide 188
  see also fluid therapy
inguinal blocks 59
inhalational anaesthetic agents 85–86
  elderly patients 108, 112
  lactic acidosis 96
inhalational analgesia (Entonox) 56, 62
inotropes
  aortic aneurysm surgery 160
  intra-operative 94
  resuscitation 89
  stress testing 20–21
  see also dobutamine; milrinone
integer logarithm risk scales 243–244
intensive care units
  acute renal failure incidence 182
  admission criteria 227–237
  blood transfusions 221–223
  elderly patients 114
  high dependency units *vs* 229
  NCEPOD recommendations 43
  patients from 78
  see also critical care
interleukin-6, blood transfusions 218
intermittent dialysis 192–193
intermittent positive pressure ventilation
  blood transfusions and weaning
    221 222
  gender on clinical risk 3
interventricular septum, pulmonary
    hypertension 149
intestinal obstruction *see* bowel obstruction
intra-aortic balloon pumps 133, 211
intracranial haemorrhage 77
intracranial pressure increase 88
intrapleural local anaesthesia 60

intravenous route
  dopamine 190
  frusemide 188
  heparin, epidural anaesthesia and 67
  nitrates 137
  opioids 56
  see also fluid therapy
intrinsic clearance, ageing 107
inulin clearance, ageing 104
iron, decreased availability 216
ischaemia, aortic aneurysm surgery
    161–162
  spinal cord 158
ischaemic heart disease *see* coronary artery
    disease; myocardial ischaemia
isoflurane 86
isoprenaline, pulmonary hypertension 151

jaundice, renal failure risk 183
junior staff
  critical care problems 233
  decisions to operate 46

ketamine 84
  sepsis 88
  shock 87
  tissue oxygen extraction 96
ketorolac, limb pain 59
kidney
  ageing 104–105, 107, 108
  blood flow *see* renal blood flow
  see also renal failure

lactic acidosis, inhalational anaesthetic
    agents 96
laparoscopy, respiratory risk 32 (Table)
laparotomy, for post-operative sepsis 175
laryngoscopy, NCEPOD recommendations
    for 43
left atrium, mitral stenosis 146–147
left ventricle
  ageing 102
  aortic regurgitation 145
  aortic stenosis 143
  central venous pressure 90
  ejection fraction 23
  end diastolic pressure 135

left ventricle (*contd*)
   radionuclide imaging 22–23
   resting function 202
leucocytosis, blood transfusions 219
leucodepleted blood transfusions 219
level of consciousness, warning of
      deterioration 235 (Table)
levels of care, Department of Health on
      227–228
limbs, pain 59
liver, ageing 105
   drug clearance 107
liver failure, renal failure 183
local anaesthesia 60
   emergency admissions 56
   peripheral nerve blocks 59
   techniques 65–75
local anaesthetic agents 68–69
   multi-modal analgesia 55
locum doctors, NCEPOD on 45
logarithm risk scales 243–244
low molecular weight heparin, epidural
      anaesthesia and 67, 68

malaria, blood transfusion risk 218
mannitol
   on kidney 188
   on reperfusion injury 162
maximum oxygen uptake 15
melanomas, gender on clinical risk 2
metabolic acidosis 96–97
   aortic aneurysm surgery 160
metabolic equivalent levels, exercise
      tolerance 15
methylxanthines, stress testing and 21
metoclopramide 168
MEWS (Modified Early Warning Score),
      critical illness 235
midazolam, shocked patients 87
milrinone
   aortic regurgitation 145–146
   mitral regurgitation 149
   pulmonary hypertension 150
miscalibration bias, risk perception 242
mitral regurgitation 141, 147–149, 208
mitral stenosis 141, 146–147, 208
   clinical risk 7–8

Modified Cardiac Risk Index 11
Modified Early Warning Score, critical illness
      235
monitoring, intra-operative 89, 90–91,
      135–136
   aortic aneurysm surgery 156
   gastrointestinal surgery 167
   valvular heart disease 142
morbid obesity
   analgesia 59
   clinical risk 31
   positive end-expiratory pressure
      ventilation 173
moribund patients, decision to operate 46
morphine 85
   algorithm controlled 57
   gastrointestinal surgery 169
   intravenous 56
mortality 246–247
   acute renal failure 194–195
   anaemia 220
   aortic aneurysms 153–154, 163
   blood transfusions 221
      ABO incompatible 220
      packed cells 217
   cardiac surgery, renal failure 183
   on critical care costs 230
   epidural anaesthesia on 72
   gastrointestinal surgery 166
   haemodynamics, peri-operative 119
   NHS Performance Indicators 42
   patient profiles 45
   risk levels 245 (Fig.)
multi-modal analgesia 55–56, 58
   multiple pain sites 60–61
multiple organ failure syndrome 117–118
   avoidance 97
murder, risk levels 244
murmurs 7
muscle relaxants 85
   respiratory risk 33
myocardial infarction
   clinical risk 5
      ACC/AHA guidelines 15
      age 5
   peri-operative 211
   prevention 119

recurrence risk 6 (Table)
surgery after 134
myocardial ischaemia 127
  aortic stenosis 143–144
  exercise stress testing 20
  haemodynamic changes causing 135
  hypothermia 81
  intra-operative detection and management
    137
  radionuclide imaging 23
myocardium
  oxygen management 134–135
    anaemia 217
  perfusion stress radionuclide imaging
    22–23, 24, 202
  revascularisation *see* coronary
    revascularisation

nasogastric tubes 168
  aortic aneurysm surgery 156
National Confidential Enquiry into
    Perioperative Deaths (NCEPOD)
    41–49
  recommendations 42–48
  statistics on elderly patients 109
  website 48
National Health Service Performance
    Indicators (NCEPOD) 42
National Lottery, probabilities 244
NCCG (non-consultant career grade
    doctors), NCEPOD on 45
NCEPOD *see* National Confidential Enquiry
    into Perioperative Deaths
Negroes, North American
  endometrial cancer 3
  prostate cancer 3
neoplasms
  ethnicity on risk 3
  recurrence, blood transfusions 170–171, 219
neostigmine, bowel anastomoses 169
neurological injury
  anaesthesia, risk levels 245 (Fig.)
  aortic cross-clamping 158
neurones, ageing 106
neuropathic pain 55
neurosurgery, NCEPOD recommendations
    for 43

neurotransmitters, ageing 106, 107
neutrophils, activated 162
nicorandil (potassium channel activator),
    pre-operative 131, 132
nicotine 30
night surgery
  avoidance 43
  clinical risk 2
nitrates *e.g.* nitroglycerin
  Charing Cross protocol 189
  intra-operative 205
  intravenous 137
  pre-operative 131, 132
  pulmonary hypertension 150
nitric oxide, pulmonary hypertension 150
nitrous oxide 86
  gastrointestinal surgery 168
non-consultant career grade doctors,
    NCEPOD on 45
non-invasive testing, coronary artery disease
    6, 18–24, 130
non-steroidal anti-inflammatory drugs
  multi-modal analgesia 55
  platelet function 67
  renal failure 183
noradrenaline 94
  hypertrophic cardiomyopathy 207
  renal failure prevention 189–190
  septic shock 95
noradrenaline (endogenous), ageing 106
normal pressure hydrocephalus, ageing 105
nucleotides, immune system stimulation 172
nutritional support, gastrointestinal surgery
    171–172

obesity
  respiratory risk 31
  see also morbid obesity
obstructive jaundice, renal failure risk 183
oesophagectomy (cardio-oesophagectomy),
    risk 247 (Table)
oliguria 180
  vs non-oliguric renal failure 187–188
omega 3 fatty acids, immune system
    stimulation 172
omeprazole 168
operating theatres, management in 77–100

operations *see* surgical procedures
opioids
 algorithm controlled 57
 elderly patients 112
 epidural anaesthesia 57, 60, 70
 gastrointestinal surgery 169
 general anaesthesia 84–85
 multi–modal analgesia 55
 respiratory depression 54, 70
 spinal analgesia 70
  on stress response 175
optimal goals (Shoemaker) 96
optimisation, peri–operative 117–125
 coronary artery disease 133–134
organ donors, colloids and 185
organ failure
 pain on 53
 peri–operative optimisation and 123
 see also multiple organ failure syndrome
orthopaedic surgery
 regional anaesthesia 74
 see also femoral neck fracture
osmolality, urine, acute renal failure 180
outreach, critical care 234
oxygen consumption
 kidney 186, 187
 peri–operative optimisation 120
 rewarming 81
oxygen debt 96–97
oxygen delivery
 anaemia 215
 critical point 220
 kidney 186, 187
 peri–operative optimisation 120, 121,
  123
oxygen demand, *vs* supply, myocardium 135
oxygen tension, arterial
 ageing 103
 clinical risk 37
oxygen therapy
 aortic aneurysm surgery 157
 elderly patients 112
  post–operative 113
oxygen transport 95–97
oxygen uptake, maximum 15
oxyhaemoglobin dissociation curve, anaemia
  216

pacing, pacemakers (cardiac) 210
packed cell transfusions *see* red blood cell
  transfusions
pain
 ageing on pathways 106
 assessment 54–55
 high dependency unit admission criteria
  231
 pathophysiology 52–53
'Pain after Surgery' (RCS/RCA) 51–52
pancuronium 85
 respiratory complications 33, 173
paracetamol, multi–modal analgesia 55
'paradoxical' bradycardia 95
parenteral nutrition 171–172
parvovirus B19, blood transfusion risk 218
patient-controlled analgesia 51, 57
 elderly patients 113
 epidural 58
  incident pain 61–62
patient positioning 79–80
 elderly patients 111
patient refusal
 epidural anaesthesia 59
 see also consent
patient selection, peri–operative optimisation
  122–123
patient transfer 78–79
penetrating injuries, permissive hypovolaemia
  93
perception of risk 239–243
percutaneous drainage, abdominal abscesses
  175
percutaneous transluminal coronary
  angioplasty 24, 25, 131, 205
perforated viscus 175
 colon 176
Performance Indicators, National Health
  Service, NCEPOD 42
perfusion stress radionuclide imaging,
  myocardial 22–23, 24, 202
peri–operative deaths *see* National
  Confidential Enquiry into
  Perioperative Deaths
peri–operative optimisation 117–125
 coronary artery disease 133–134
peripheral nerve blocks 59

peripheral vascular disease, clinical risk and 8–9

permissive hypovolaemia 93

personnel *see* staff

pethidine, gastrointestinal surgery 169

pH, intramucosal 170
    stomach 4, 92, 123, 170

pharmacodynamics, pharmacokinetics, ageing 107–108

physicians, NCEPOD on availability 47

'physiological police' 235

physiotherapy, on respiratory complications 174

plane crashes, availability bias in risk perception 240–241

Plasmodium spp., blood transfusion risk 218

platelet function, epidural anaesthesia 67

positioning *see* patient positioning

positive end-expiratory pressure ventilation, morbid obesity 173

positive framing 243

Possum scoring system 13, 232
    NCEPOD on 46

post-mortem review, NCEPOD on 47–48

post-operative care
    aortic surgery 162–163
    coronary artery disease 137–138, 211
    elderly patients 113–114
    heart failure 207, 211
    high dependency unit admission criteria 232
    intensive care unit admission criteria 232–233
    NCEPOD on critical care 47
    see also analgesia

post-operative forced expiratory volume '1', predicted 36

post-operative hypothermia 80–81

potassium channel activator, nicorandil, pre-operative 131, 132

predicted post-operative forced expiratory volume '1' 36

pre-operative assessment
    ACC/AHA guidelines 13–15
    aortic aneurysm surgery 154–155
    vs clinical risk 25
    coronary artery disease 128–132

elderly patients 109–110
    heart 199–203
    NCEPOD on 45–47
    respiratory risk 33–37

pressure gradients
    aortic stenosis 142
    mitral stenosis 146

pressure sores, epidural anaesthesia 61

probabilities, risk 240
    communicating on 243–244

prognostic gradient, stress testing 202

prokinetic agents, gastrointestinal 168

prolactin, dopamine on 191

propofol 84
    sepsis 87–88

prostacycline, pulmonary hypertension 150

prostate cancer, North American Negroes 3

prosthetic heart valves 208–209

protein binding, ageing 107

proton pump blockers 168

PTCA (coronary angioplasty) 24, 25, 131, 205

publication bias, risk assessment 240–241

pulmonary artery catheters 90–91, 136, 137
    aortic aneurysm surgery 159
    valvular heart disease 142
        mitral regurgitation 149
        mitral stenosis 147

pulmonary capillary wedge pressure 90
    peri-operative optimisation 121

pulmonary function testing 34–36

pulmonary hypertension 149–151

pulmonary volume reduction surgery, pulmonary function testing 35–36

quality of care, critical care problems 233–234

race, on clinical risk 3

radiographic contrast media *see* X-ray contrast media

radionuclide myocardial perfusion stress imaging 22–23, 24, 202

railway accidents, risk levels 244

rapid sequence induction
    aortic aneurysm surgery 157
    cricoid pressure 168

red blood cell transfusions
  bactericidal permeability increasing
    protein 218
  cancer recurrence 170–171
  problems 217
reflexes, ageing 106
regional anaesthesia 65–66
  anticoagulants 66–68
  aspirin 67, 112
  coronary artery disease 137
  elderly patients 74, 111, 112
  intercurrent disease 72–74
  stress response to surgery 71, 174–175
  see also epidural anaesthesia; spinal
    anaesthesia
remifentanil 84–85
renal blood flow
  anaesthesia 185
  aortic cross-clamping 159
  vs perfusion pressure 189–190
  sepsis 186
renal failure 179–197
  elderly patients 108, 183
  high dependency unit admission criteria
    231
  local anaesthesia in 73–74
renal insufficiency, definition 179
renal replacement therapies 192–194
renal tubular function, ageing 104
renin, ageing 105
reperfusion injury, aortic aneurysm surgery
  161–162
respiratory centre, local anaesthetic agents 69
respiratory depression
  epidural anaesthesia 58, 70
  opioids 54, 70
respiratory rate, warning of deterioration 235
respiratory system
  ageing 103–104, 108
  clinical risk, general anaesthesia 33
  complications 29–39
  epidural anaesthesia 71
  gastrointestinal surgery 172–174
  high dependency unit admission criteria
    231
  local anaesthesia 73
resting function, left ventricle 202

resuscitation 89
  aortic aneurysm surgery 156
    progressive resistance 161–162
Revised Cardiac Risk Index 11–13
rewarming 81
rhabdomyolysis
  bicarbonate for 187
  mannitol 188
  renal failure 183
rheumatic valve disease 143
right ventricle
  mitral stenosis 146
  pulmonary hypertension 149
risk 239–247
  cardiac 4–25, 129, 199–200
  of critical illness developing 234
  factors 1–28
  gastrointestinal surgery 165–166
  general anaesthesia 245 (Fig.)
  indicators (Shoemaker) 118
  stratification 4–5, 14, 15, 18
  valvular heart disease 141
risk-benefit analysis 246–247
rocuronium 85
routes of administration
  emergency analgesia 56
  see also intravenous route; subcutaneous
    heparin
Royal College of Anaesthetists
  'Pain after Surgery' 51–52
  on supervision 45
Royal College of Surgeons, 'Pain after
  Surgery' 51–52
Royal Society, definitions of hazard and risk
  239

saline infusion, metabolic acidosis from 97
salvage devices, blood transfusions 161
scales
  pain assessment 55
  see also scoring systems
scheduled surgery, NCEPOD definition
  48
scoring systems
  clinical risk 9–13
  Early Warning Score, critical illness 235
  see also scales

senior help requests 44, 46
sepsis
    abdomen 173
    acute renal failure 181
    anaesthetic agents 87–88
    epidural anaesthesia 60
    gastrointestinal surgery 175
    gender on clinical risk 2
    haemofiltration trial 193
    inotropes and vasopressors 94–95
    kidney blood flow 186
    peri-operative optimisation and 123
    renal failure 181, 185
    staff availability on clinical risk 1
septum, interventricular, pulmonary
        hypertension 149
sestamibi 22
severity of risk 241
severity scoring systems
    clinical risk 9–13
    intensive care unit admission criteria 232
sevoflurane 85
shock
    cardiogenic 94
    general anaesthesia 86–87
    haemorrhagic *vs* traumatic 95–96
    inotropes and vasopressors 94–95
Shoemaker, W.C., risk indicators 118
site of surgery *see* anatomical site of surgery
skin, patient positioning 80
sleep apnoea, analgesia 59
smoking, respiratory risk 30
sodium
    aged kidney 105
    urine, acute renal failure 180
spinal anaesthesia
    aortic stenosis 144
    benefits 71–72
    complications 66, 73
    elderly patients 112–113
    haematoma risk 68
    opioids 70
        on stress response 175
    risk levels 245 (Fig.)
    on stress response to surgery 174–175
spinal cord ischaemia, aortic cross-clamping
        158

spine
    elderly patients 112
    protection 80
splanchnic hypoperfusion 117
staff
    clinical risk and 1–2
    critical care problems 233
    decisions to operate 46
    NCEPOD recommendations 43–45
sternotomy, pain 60
stomach
    full, gastrointestinal surgery 167–168
    intramucosal pH 4, 92, 123, 170
storage lesions (of blood products) 217
stress response to surgery
    gastrointestinal surgery 174–175
    regional anaesthesia 71, 174–175
stress testing 19–24, 130
    exercise 20, 23–24, 130, 201–202
    prognostic gradients 202
ST segment monitoring, computerised 137,
        211
subcutaneous heparin, epidural anaesthesia
        and 67–68
subendocardial ischaemia
    aortic stenosis 143–144
    radionuclide imaging 23
supervision, NCEPOD on 44, 45
supranormal values, peri-operative
        optimisation for 120, 121, 123
surface area (valve), aortic stenosis 142
surgeons, as risk factor 1–2
surgical procedures
    high dependency unit admission criteria
        232
    risk stratification of 16–17
suxamethonium 85
sympathetic blockade
    epidural anaesthesia 66
    haemodynamics, elderly patients 106, 113

tachycardia
    mitral stenosis 147
    myocardial ischaemia 135
    pulmonary hypertension 150
technetium-99m, myocardial perfusion stress
        imaging 22

temperature, warning of deterioration 235
thallium-201, myocardial perfusion stress
        imaging 22, 24, 202
theatres *see* emergency theatres; operating
        theatres
thiopentone 83–84, 87
    animal studies 87
third heart sound 7
third space fluid loss, gastrointestinal surgery
        170
thoracic cage compliance, ageing 103
thoracic surgery
    post-operative pain 60
    respiratory risk 32 (Table)
thromboembolism
    epidural anaesthesia 71
    NCEPOD on prophylaxis 47
thyroxine 192
tidal volume
    ageing 104
    ventilation, on respiratory complications
        173
total parenteral nutrition 171–172
tracheostomy 82
training
    ALERT course 236
    Clinical Negligence Scheme for Trusts on
        45
    need for 1
tramadol, multi-modal analgesia 56
transfer of patients 78–79
transferrin deficiency 216
transfusions *see* blood (product) transfusions
transoesophageal echocardiography
    myocardial ischaemia 137
    valvular heart disease 142
trauma 77
    haemofiltration trial 193
    hypothermia 80
    peri-operative optimisation 121
    permissive hypovolaemia 93
    staff availability on surgical risk 1
traumatic shock, haemorrhagic shock *vs*
        95–96
Trypanosoma cruzi, blood transfusion risk 218
tubular necrosis, acute 180
tubuloglomerular feedback 186

tumours
    ethnicity on risk 3
    recurrence, blood transfusions 170–171,
        219

United Kingdom, United States, bowel
        cancer surgery volumes 1–2
uraemia 192
urea measurement, renal failure 181
urgent admission, urgent surgery, NCEPOD
        definitions 48
urinary catheterisation, aortic aneurysm
        surgery 156
urine
    electrolytes, acute renal failure 180
    output, warning of deterioration
        235 (Table)
    timed collections 181

valve surface area, aortic stenosis 142
valvular heart disease 141–149, 207–209
    clinical risk and 7–8
    prosthetic valves 208–209
vascular surgery
    anaemia, morbidity 220
    gender on clinical risk 3
    peri-operative optimisation 120–121
    renal failure risk 183
vasoconstriction, dopamine 190
vasoconstrictors
    cocaine 69
    local anaesthesia 69–70
vasodilatation, rewarming 81
vasodilators
    coronary, stress testing 21
    local anaesthetic agents as 69
    pulmonary hypertension 150
vasopressors
    intra-operative 94–95
    resuscitation 89
vecuronium 85
    respiratory risk 33
veins, ageing 102
venovenous haemofiltration, continuous
        192–194
ventilation 82–83
    blood transfusions and weaning 221–222

patient transfer 78
tidal volume on respiratory complications
173
see also intermittent positive pressure
ventilation
VIP system, resuscitation 89
vital capacity, ageing 103
volatile agents *see* inhalational anaesthetic
agents
volume (clinical), *vs* risk 1–2
volume loading (fluids)
gastrointestinal surgery 170
intra-operative 92–93
vulnerability, risk perception 241

ward care
critical care problems 233

epidural anaesthesia 58
patients from 77
warming
aortic aneurysm surgery 156
gastrointestinal surgery 167
rewarming 81
workload (clinical volume), *vs* risk 1–2
wounds
local anaesthetic infiltration 60, 95
metabolic activity of 96

xanthines (methylxanthines), stress testing
and 21
X-ray contrast media
acute renal failure 182, 184, 187, 188
dopamine and 191